The Essential Guide to Becoming a Staff Nurse

T0201440

To staff nurses, past, present and future

The Essential Guide to Becoming a Staff Nurse

Ian Peate

WILEY Blackwell

This edition first published 2016 © by John Wiley & Sons, Ltd

Registered office: John Wiley & Sons, Ltd, The Atrium, Southern Gate, Chichester, West Sussex, PO19 8SQ, UK

Editorial offices: 9600 Garsington Road, Oxford, OX4 2DQ, UK

The Atrium, Southern Gate, Chichester, West Sussex, PO19 8SQ, UK

1606 Golden Aspen Drive, Suites 103 and 104, Ames, Iowa 50010, USA

For details of our global editorial offices, for customer services and for information about how to apply for permission to reuse the copyright material in this book please see our website at www.wiley.com/wiley-blackwell.

The right of the author to be identified as the author of this work has been asserted in accordance with the UK Copyright, Designs and Patents Act 1988.

Library of Congress Cataloging-in-Publication Data applied for.

A catalogue record for this book is available from the British Library.

Wiley also publishes its books in a variety of electronic formats. Some content that appears in print may not be available in electronic books.

Cover image: Getty images/466458497/by sturti

Set in 8.5/12pt, MeridienLTStd by SPi Global, Chennai, India.

Printed in Singapore by C.O.S. Printers Pte Ltd

1   2016

Contents

About the Author

Ian Peate EN(G) RGN DipN (Lond) RNT BEd (Hons) MA (Lond) LLM

Ian began his nursing career in 1981 at Central Middlesex Hospital, becoming an enrolled nurse working in an intensive care unit. He later undertook 3 years of student nurse training at Central Middlesex and Northwick Park Hospitals, becoming a staff nurse and then a charge nurse. He has worked in nurse education since 1989. His key areas of interest are nursing practice and theory, men's health, sexual health and HIV. Ian has published widely; he is Professor of Nursing, Editor in Chief of the *British Journal of Nursing* and Head of School at the School of Health Studies, Gibraltar.

Editor in Chief *British Journal of Nursing*,
Head of School
School of Health Studies
Gibraltar

Acknowledgements

I would like to thank my partner Jussi Lahtinen for his ongoing support and encouragement, Mrs Frances Cohen for her continued help and assistance, Anthony Peate who contributed to the illustrations and the library staff at St Bernard's Hospital, Gibraltar.

Preface

Becoming a staff nurse brings with it a lot of mixed emotions, responsibilities and a salary. Three years of blood, sweat, tears and laughter have led to this position, but still your journey is not over as you become truly a lifelong learner.

The transition from student nurse to staff nurse takes place overnight, from being a student nurse and then a registered nurse with a personal identification number from the Nursing and Midwifery Council (NMC) and then there is the change from being responsible to being accountable; for some this can be daunting. Some may suggest the transition takes 3 years, from the day you commenced your education. The text aims to facilitate the transitional process.

Contemporary nursing practice is constantly changing and evolving. Historically, nursing has been offered at certificate level and then diploma level and now entry to the professional register can only occur if the registrant has been educated to degree level. Since September 2013 all pre-registration nursing programmes leading to registration have been at a minimum undergraduate degree level. Throughout all the changes the length of the programmes has remained at 3 years.

The title Nurse is a title that is protected in law; no person is allowed to purport to be a nurse unless his or her name appears on the professional register and no person can practice nursing unless his or her name has been entered onto the professional register. Entry to the professional register can only occur when the standards that the NMC have set for education have been met. You have met those standards (exacting standards) and your name is on the professional register. You have made it, be proud and uphold the standards of the profession, congratulations!

There has been a massive reorganisation of health and social service provision and there have been a number of high-profile cases concerning nursing and nurses reported in the media. All of this has had an impact on the role and function of the newly registered nurse – the staff nurse.

The world continues to change and in response to this the provision of nursing services has also needed to change. Nurses are now working in a variety of health and social care sectors that had hitherto been unheard of. This text takes into account the direction for nursing as detailed in policy and practice, identifying the changes necessary to the way nurses work and to their roles, responsibilities, educational and developmental requirements in order to deliver safe, competent and compassionate patient-centred nursing services. The text is suited to the community setting, primary and acute care with an emphasis upon the adult field of nursing; however, the broad principles can be applied across all fields.

Each chapter begins with an aim and a set of objectives helping the reader pre-plan for what is to come and to understand the rationale for the discrete yet intertwined chapters. Text layout has been given much thought, aiming to ensure that it is user friendly and engaging. There are 10 chapters. Inspiration is provided throughout the text at appropriate intervals offering the reader practical hints and tips, where you are asked to consider specific issues. You will be asked to carry out a variety of exercises along the way, where the author hands over to the staff nurse.

An evidence base is used to support discussion. Reference and referral to organisations such as the Royal College of Nursing, the NMC, UNISON, National Institute for Health and Care Excellence, Scottish Intercollegiate Guidelines Network and other appropriate organisations is made. Referral to the revised 2015 Code of Conduct (Nursing and Midwifery Council, 2015) and other guidance issued by the regulator has been included.

The text will help support you as you endeavour to offer safe, effective, evidence-based and patient-centred care, with the patient at the heart of all that you do. The information provided will help generate confidence and understanding. The book provides you with material that will help you to consolidate your three-year education programme as you make the transition from student to staff nurse, the autonomous and accountable practitioner.

It is anticipated that it will help you appreciate how your role and function must change now that your name has been entered on the professional register. The text does not aim to provide you with a repertoire of skills that will enable you to perform clinical procedures; it should be seen more as a resource, an aide memoir, as you are about to begin your work as a registered nurse.

The text is designed to be used as a reference text, compact enough to be carried in the pocket, small enough to be put in a bag and referred to throughout the day, at home, on the train or at work. It is not intended to be read from cover to cover in one sitting; it should be used as a guide, a reference. This text provides you with details concerning the theory of leadership and management and teamwork as well as offering helpful hints and tips about the 'doing' aspect of the role; the key principles are provided in one text, avoiding the need to visit several texts.

Reference

Nursing and Midwifery Council (2015) "The Code. Professional Standards of Practice and Behaviour for Nurses and Midwives" http://www.nmc-uk.org/Documents/NMC-Publications/NMC-Code-A5-FINAL.pdf last (accessed February 2015).

CHAPTER 1

Getting the job you want

Aim

The aim of this chapter is to help you get the job you want.

Objectives

By the end of this chapter you will be able to:
1. Give some consideration to your future career prospects
2. Have further understanding of your role as a staff nurse
3. Read a job description critically
4. Put together your curriculum vitae (CV)
5. Understand how to complete an application for a job
6. Prepare for interview

Introduction

CONGRATULATIONS STAFF NURSE! Well done, you did it! Three years of hard labour, blood, sweat and for sure plenty of tears, and your name now appears on the professional register. OK, enough of the celebrations; it is time to get that job you really want.

In some areas jobs are hard to find and the competition can be stiff. You have to stand out above the crowd but you will need more than your good looks, wit and humour. The way to get the job that you want is to prepare, prepare and prepare; oh, and did I say prepare?

This opening chapter will consider the role of the staff nurse and some of the issues that can impact on the nurse's role and function. It is essential that you give serious consideration to where you want to be in 5 years' time (a common question used at interviews); so you must have an understanding of the various

The Essential Guide to Becoming a Staff Nurse, First Edition. Ian Peate.
© 2016 John Wiley & Sons, Ltd. Published 2016 by John Wiley & Sons, Ltd.

career options available to you. This chapter cannot do this for you; you have to do this but, be bold, think wide and far. Your registration is in effect your passport to the rest of the word – the world really is your oyster.

Application by curriculum vitae (CV) is becoming more popular; the chapter provides pointers on CVs. You must not forget however that the completion of a standard application form (electronic or hand written) is still very much used, particularly in the NHS.

There are sections in the chapter that help you read and understand a job description, encouraging you to look at it in a critical light. When you have considered your career trajectory, you have critically analysed the job description, tailored your CV to reflect the person specification and completed the application and have been invited for interview; at this point you really do have to talk the talk and walk the walk. There are hints and tips towards the end of the chapter that will help you prepare for interview.

The role of the staff nurse

Over the years the role of the staff nurse (the registered nurse) has changed and will continue to change and evolve. The changes are often the result of professional, statutory requirements as well as the demands made by the public on nurses and health services. Nurses are members of the multidisciplinary team, often acting as a pivot, the coordinator of care, particularly in the health care setting. The team will have common goals but each with their own different roles to perform. The Royal College of Nursing, RCN (2013) has defined various roles within what it calls the nursing family (see table 1.1).

The multidisciplinary/inter-relational working arrangements of the various members of the nursing team can be found in figure 1.1.

The Health and Social Care Act 2012

This Act has introduced changes for the delivery of health and social care and has been hailed at the biggest changes to the NHS since the system was set up in 1948. A summary of some aspects of the Act is detailed in table 1.2. The Health and Social Care Act (the Act) is divided into 12 parts and is only relevant to England.

When the Act was introduced, primary care trusts and strategic health authorities were abolished as part of the radical restructuring of the health service; new health and well-being boards have been established with the aim of improving integration between the NHS and local authority services. Clinical commissioning groups have taken over commissioning from primary care trusts

Table 1.1 The nursing team – roles.

Registered nurses	Assistant practitioners	Health care assistants
• Use their specific knowledge to make clinical judgements in order to assess the needs of the people they care for • Prescribe, appropriately delegate and supervise nursing care • Are accountable practitioners as well as being accountable for the care that they have delegated to others	• Support the work of a variety of registered professionals, crossing professional boundaries • Makes judgements using a comparative approach • Plan their own work in line with accepted protocols and standard operating procedures • Can undertake the routine supervision of others	• Have nursing tasks delegated to them by the registered nurse and are supervised when providing care to people • Work within and are guided by protocols that have been set • Undertake the performance of tasks that are commensurate with their level of assessed competence • Have responsibility to inform the person delegating tasks if they do not have the competence to undertake it

Source: Adapted from Royal College of Nursing (2003, 2013) and Skills for Health (2010).

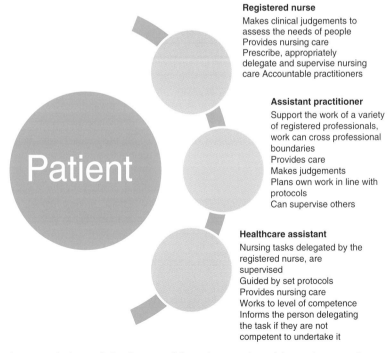

Registered nurse

Makes clinical judgements to assess the needs of people
Provides nursing care
Prescribe, appropriately delegate and supervise nursing care Accountable practitioners

Assistant practitioner

Support the work of a variety of registered professionals, work can cross professional boundaries
Provides care
Makes judgements
Plans own work in line with protocols
Can supervise others

Healthcare assistant

Nursing tasks delegated by the registered nurse, are supervised
Guided by set protocols
Provides nursing care
Works to level of competence
Informs the person delegating the task if they are not competent to undertake it

Figure 1.1 The inter-relational aspects of the various members of the nursing team. Source: Adapted from Royal College of Nursing (2013).

Table 1.2 A summary of some aspects of the 2012 Health and Social Care Act.

- The health service in England incorporating duties of the Secretary of State for Health and new commissioning measures
- Further provisions about public health as well as direction on the cooperation of bodies with functions relating to public health
- Regulation of health and adult social care services (particularly Monitor), competition issues, licensing, pricing, health special administration and financial assistance in special administration cases
- NHS foundation trusts and NHS trusts
- Public involvement and local government concerning HealthWatch at national (England) and local levels
- Primary care services
- Regulation of health and social care workers
- The National Institute for Health and Care Excellence (NICE), including a slight name change from the National Institute for Health and Clinical Excellence
- Information concerning health and adult social care services
- Abolition of some public bodies, such as, the Appointments Commission, the National Patient Safety Agency and the Alcohol Education and Research Council
- Miscellaneous, including information relating to births and deaths, duties to cooperate and supervised community treatment under the Mental Health Act 1983
- Final provisions, comprising financial provisions and commencement of a consultation with Scottish Ministers

and are working with the new NHS Commissioning Board. Monitor, a new regulator has been established to regulate providers of NHS services in the interests of patients and to prevent anticompetitive behaviour. The voices of those who use services have been strengthened with the setting up of a new national body, HealthWatch, and local HealthWatch organisations. Public Health England, a new body, is leading on public health nationally and local authorities do this at a local level.

These changes to the provision have had significant impact on the ways in which nurses work as well as on whom they work with. Having insight and being able to demonstrate this insight can help you at interview as you will be expected to be able to show an understanding of how the NHS is run and how the nurse contributes to its success.

Being up to date and demonstrating this at interview means not only being on top of contemporary practice issues but also having an all-round understanding of the politics of health and social care. You will only be able to confidently state facts with regard to how the provision of care is delivered at micro and macro levels and what has an impact on this if you have done your homework.

Things to consider

Take some time and think about the people who may be interviewing you for this your dream job. They are more than likely highly educated and in positions of seniority; they have seen so many changes over the years in many forms. They have seen changes made to the roles and function of nurses, they are looking for someone who knows what contemporary nursing is all about and they want you to be able to tell them what the drivers are behind role change. Do your homework and dig deep; be ready to discuss the politics behind the role.

The job description

A staff nurse's job is a staff nurse's job anywhere – wrong, and this is why it is essential that you are critical of the job description. At first glance according to Tremayne (2009) all jobs seem to offer the same things – excitement, challenge and flexibility. This is done in order to try and make their job stand out.

During your nursing studies you will have been asked as a senior student in your academic work to 'critically analyse'. The skills that you have developed during your studies will now come into play with regard to the job description.

Critical analysis does not mean being negative; it requires you to be objective with regard to the job description and look for the good and not so good aspects. You have to be focused and try to avoid being subjective; it is so easy to do this when you are so keen to get a job. What you want is the job of your dreams.

A job description is an outline of a job; it can be anywhere from a few sentences to a few pages long. Being able to quickly and correctly analyse the job description can help you search for employment more effectively.

Often job seekers apply for jobs based only on the job title. Job titles are usually 'general', for example, 'staff nurse'; what is most important is to look at the key responsibilities to make sure that your skill set really matches the role. If you do not have some relevant skills, then there is little chance they will call you forward for interview. Spend more time reading the information as opposed to focusing on the job.

You should avoid giving the selector (those that sift the applications) the impression that you are applying for every advert out there regardless of whether you have the relevant skill set or experience for that position. Having read the job description in a critical way you will come across as being a person who knows what the potential employer is looking for as opposed to casting a very wide net. The people doing the hiring want to be sure that the applicant has clearly read the job description (see table 1.3).

Table 1.3 The job description critically analysed.

- Take time to evaluate your own job experience and skills before evaluating the job description. It is essential that you know your applicable skills, experience and education level
- Print out the job description. Using a highlighter pen underline or highlight important qualifications. You can also copy and paste the description into a word processor document and highlight lines if you prefer
- Identify the job location. This should be listed at the top. Do not apply for the job if you are not available to work in that area. There are some positions that may specify that they will require you to work at various locations (locally or nationally)
- Identify and highlight the education required for the post. This is often listed as diploma, bachelor's degree, master's degree, certification or another form of qualification that may be related to the speciality. Decide if you qualify based on the education level
- Highlight the skills necessary for the job. This could be written in a list or in prose format. If it is listed in sentences or paragraph form, list the skills on another piece of paper, underlining each skill that you possess. Look for skills associated with the use of information technology, interpersonal skills, familiarity with technical terms, experience in specific areas, fields (i.e. child, mental health, learning disability or adult), problem-solving skills, physical demands and more
- Identify and highlight the experience required for the job. Pay attention to language when looking at experience. If 3 years is listed as a requirement, the employer is likely to be strict; however, if 3 years is listed as a 'desired qualification' then it may not be strictly necessary
- Identify the daily activities that are involved in the job. Highlight hours, specific duties and daily tasks. Make sure you can complete these tasks prior to applying
- Go through the job description looking for specific requirements. Some positions may require that you are to work on internal rotation. If you cannot fulfil these requirements, then do not apply for the job. They are non-negotiable
- Highlight the salary and other forms of compensation. Near the end of the job description, there is usually a salary or grade stated. Sometimes, the description will say depends on experience, which means that the salary is negotiable based on how well you fulfil the qualifications
- Decide if you fulfil the education, experience, skills and various requirements listed in the job posting. If you do decide to move forward in the application process write a covering letter and adjust your CV to address your applicable qualifications. It is essential that you write a covering letter and a CV that addresses each job you apply for specifically. This demonstrates that you have researched the organisation
- Identify the steps that are necessary to apply for the job. Many job descriptions state clearly where a CV, a covering letter or inquiries can be sent. Highlight the deadline to apply and ensure that you adhere strictly to that deadline

Applying for a job can be easy, but applying for the right job is not always easy when you have to match the job profile. If you have questions about the description, find out more by calling the organisation. Only apply if you think you can actually do the job.

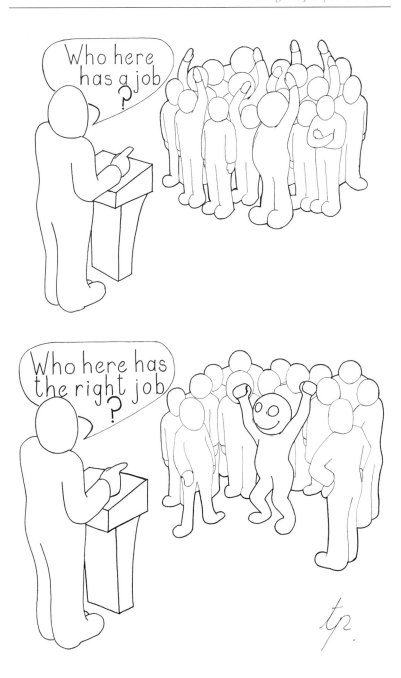

Over to you staff nurse

The anatomy of a job description

Choose a job description for a job that interests you and complete the following list:

1 What is the purpose of the position (the reasons for the position's existence)?
2 What is the position on offer (title, grade/salary, department, directorate and so on)?
3 What are the essential functions associated with the position (the tasks critical to the position)?
4 Periodic functions (tasks that are not essential, but are part of the job description)?
5 List the minimum qualifications (education, NMC registration required, experience).
6 What are the required behaviours (attention to detail, ability to learn)?
7 Describe the working conditions (description of the physical requirements, environmental issues).
8 Any supervision needed (how the job is supervised, whether you are expected to work independently)?
9 Miscellaneous 'Other tasks as assigned' (what are these).
   Having dissected the job description:
• Can you do the job?
• Do you still want it?

The application form

Most employers will require all applicants, regardless of the job applied for, to complete a job application form. You have filled in an application before (and in some instances on many occasions) so this is nothing new to you, but it will be different. It is essential that you tailor the application to the job on offer, hence the need to ensure that you fully understand the detail within the job description.

There are a number of organisations (e.g. trusts) who have their own application forms, and they do this for a reason. They want you to answer certain questions often related to the specific needs of the organisation and the people they offer their service to. Each organisation's working environment is very different and you need to decide if this is the environment you are looking for.

Ensure that you give full and focused answers when responding to the questions on the application form. As obvious as this may sound many people fail to make the link between what the job requires and what they have to offer.

The person selecting or sifting the applications often have two piles – 'proceed and invite' or 'reject'; they are busy people, and they need you to tell them that you have the relevant skills for the position being offered and these skills are commensurate with the job. If this is your first application for a staff nurse's job in a surgical unit you need to speak about your experiences as a student in a surgical area – what it is that has made you want to come back to that area? Do not tell the prospective employer on the application form that you 'like to do dressings'; you need to do much more convincing than that.

Things to consider

It is important for your job application to be complete, correct (no errors) and accurate. Take a photocopy of the original application form and use it for a couple of practice runs so that when you come to completing and presenting the final one it will be perfect.

Table 1.4 provides a list of hints and tips associated with filling in the application form.

Table 1.4 Some hints and tips concerning the application form.

- Read the application through first; this gives a flavour of what it is they will be asking of you
- Ensure that you have all of the information to hand, for example, dates addresses and so on
- Be sure to complete all requested information. Do not leave anything blank. If any of the responses asked for are not applicable then write 'not applicable' in the space
- Adhere to instructions, write clearly and neatly, using black ink or if instructed to do so make the application online or word process
- Check for spelling and grammatical errors. Proofread your job application form before turning it in and also ask someone else to proofread it for you
- If asked to complete a section chronologically, for example, list your most recent job first when completing employment information. List your most recent education first. Include schools, colleges and training institutions and universities
- If you are required to provide details of referees do so but, ensure you have asked the permission of the person/people you are citing to act as a referee
- Check the application form for any omission/oversights
- Do not forget to sign and date your application

You will be asked about criminal convictions on the application form; you must make any declaration that relates to clinical convictions. Good character will be assessed by the provision of two references. You should use your University for one and a clinician for the other, seeking their permission prior to putting their name down. You will be required to complete an occupational health risk/assessment form.

The personal statement

The personal statement is your opportunity to impress a future employer. Sometimes, there are word restrictions applied to the personal statement and as such you may only have a few hundred words; if you get this right then you are on your way to being invited to interview.

When constructing your personal statement you should remember that the prospective employer is looking for a person who is passionate about the job on offer, not just anyone who wants any job. The personal statement provides you with an opportunity to share with your future employer how keen you are about the position they are offering without them even seeing you.

The personal statement if written well is all about setting yourself apart from the rest of the people who are applying for the position, your opportunity to show that you are the ideal candidate. The job description tells you what the employer is looking for. Go through the job description and make a list of examples that show why and how you could fulfil each prerequisite.

When you have written the personal statement then it must be checked. Check your spelling. Did you demonstrate the ways in which you have met all the necessary competencies in the job description? Have you said why you want the job? Did you read it back to yourself aloud to ensure it makes sense? Ask someone else to check it.

You should keep it simple – you are not expected to write an essay and the prospective employer will not want to read one. Ensure the points being made are concise, demonstrate enthusiasm and professionalism.

The curriculum vitae

It is common practice for employing organisations to ask potential candidates to not only submit a completed application form but to also provide them with an up-to-date CV. Your CV is your personal marketing tool (RCN, 2005); this should be used to demonstrate to a potential employer that you have the skills and professional, educational and personal experience required to undertake

---

Things to consider

General tips to help create a CV

- Use 'action' words, for example, 'developed', 'organised', 'led', 'initiated', 'produced'.
- Do not use the pronoun 'I'.
- Provide an explanation for any gaps in your paid employment.
- Include any achievements you have gained through voluntary work or student activity, for example, set rep.
- Do not exceed two pages.
- If you have a lot of experience, summarise positions held more than 10 years ago.
- If you have published a number of articles, select the most important ones, summarising the others.
- Use good quality white paper.
- Do not use too many font styles.
- Ornate typefaces and borders are not required.
- Use black font colour.
- Do not include a photograph.
- Abbreviations that are not easily recognised should be avoided.
- Only include contact details for referees if you are happy for them to be contacted.
- Enclose a covering letter highlighting the main points of your CV and how they relate to the post you are applying for.
- Always ask for another person to proofread your CV for any errors.
- Seek constructive feedback to determine if it is easy to read and if it makes a positive impact.

---

the position you are applying for. A CV can be used for a range of purposes and in this instance when you have been asked to enclose a CV along with a standard application form.

When preparing to write your CV begin by making a list of your experience and posts held, beginning with the most recent (these include post held prior to your nurse education). List the date of employment, name of the employer, your job title, the responsibilities and your main achievements for each of the posts held.

Make a list of the courses you have undertaken and the qualifications gained; work chronologically. Include the dates and the names of the educational establishments. List any professional activities such as any articles that you have published, papers you have presented at conferences, membership of professional groups and so on.

It is recognised that there is no single perfect format to be used for the construction of a CV. The CV should be logical, clear and concise; you should emphasise your strengths. Table 1.5 provides key components that should be included in your CV.

Table 1.5 Key components of a CV.

- Personal details: Your name, address, preferred contact telephone number and email address
- Opening statement: Write a couple of sentences summarising your personal and professional qualities. Include two or three major professional achievements in the statement if you have a lot of experience
- Experience: Start this section with your most recent post, listing dates, position(s) held and the name of the employer. Provide three or four key responsibilities held at your most recent posts (even as a student) and two or three major achievements that are relevant to the position being applied for. Go through the job description and person specification in order to do this
- Qualifications: Provide details of your professional qualifications and education to date. Include your NMC pin number and expiry date
- Professional activities: Provide a list of articles published, membership of professional groups and any papers delivered at conferences
- Personal: You can include extra information, your interests, but only in general terms and only if relevant to the job. Also include whether you hold a driving licence

Source: Adapted from RCN (2005).

On paper, this is your chance to sell yourself and indicate what type of nurse you are, that you are a knowledgeable doer, that you are a kind person, compassionate and caring. In order to do this you will have to use emotive words and should not be afraid to say how passionate you are about your work.

Psychometric testing

More and more organisations are including psychometric testing (sometimes called personality or aptitude tests) and an assessment of the candidate's ability to calculate as part of the interviewing process (sometimes these tests are done prior to interview and the candidate is only then invited to proceed to interview if they are successful in the supplementary tests).

Personality tests are used to help determine how your personality relates to your choice of job, so they are important tests. An aptitude test can provide an indication of which jobs match which personality and which careers a person might have an aptitude for (they are not however fail proof). These types of tests can help assess job applicants for conscientiousness, extroversion or other traits that can be useful in helping to enhance an already established team, to forging a successful career – alternatively, to cause a derailment.

The questions are seldom straightforward, nor are the answers. There is an element of psychology involved in the setting of the questions. Applicants may try to give answers they think the organisation wants to hear. Psychometric testing is not asking you to give right answers – they are asking for you to just be yourself.

The majority of psychometric tests are completed online. Some tests enable you to save your answers and return to complete the test at a later stage; others are timed. Check if you can go back and adjust an answer before you begin a test; there are some tests that do not allow you to go back to a question once you have moved on.

As expected there are various types of psychometric tests. Personality tests aim to identify a personal type. This often takes the form of paired items or pictures and you are asked to choose a preference. For example, would you rather read a book or go to a party?

Aptitude or ability tests are those that have been designed to assess your reasoning or cognitive ability. These tests usually include:

- Verbal tests
- Numerical tests
- Spatial reasoning
- Subject/role-specific tests.

Things to consider

Preparing for the tests:

The personality test:
- Practise using tests so that you are familiar with the style being used and the format of questions.
- Answer questions honestly; do not try to guess what the 'right' answer is.

  To prepare for an aptitude test:
- Practise as many tests as you can.
- Try to determine what particular tests are being used for nursing or health care-related jobs.

  Remember, there are no right or wrong answers in personality tests, and aptitude tests are generally used as a starting point for recruitment. When taking these tests ensure that you:
- Read the instructions carefully
- Work through questions quickly and accurately
- Do not try to guess the right answer
- Answer honestly
- Practise so that you are not distracted by the way the questions have been formatted or the style used
- Pay attention to what you are being asked but do not dwell for too long; if you are unsure move on to the next question.

There are several career aptitude tests and assessments available online that can help you determine what type of job matches your career interests and aptitude as well as helping you to prepare to undertake one, if this is a part of the interview process.

Numeracy screening

The majority of health care organisations are now requiring all applications for new staff nurses posts to sit a numeracy test (many also require you to sit a literacy test). There is no standard test (i.e. one that is used across the country); each organisation will have their own test(s) and you may be required to attend an assessment centre to sit the tests.

Some of the questions in the test may seem to be rather basic however; standards of numeracy in most adults in the United Kingdom are poor regardless of their highest qualification. Candidates are required to demonstrate a minimum threshold score on the selection day if they are to progress to the interview stage. The organisation inviting you to interview will send you details of any pre-assessments that you will be required to undertake.

Things to consider

If you anticipate difficulty with the numeracy test the BBC have a site http://www.bbc.co.uk/skillswise; this site Skillswise has been set up for adults to use with regard to Maths and English. This is a free to access website with worksheets that can be printed off along with factsheets and online games, videos and quizzes.

The Standardised Numeracy Assessment Process (SNAP) aims to standardise the approach to dealing with the assessment of numeracy. The SNAP service provides numeracy assessment and education to health care and educational organisations across England. There are open source materials freely available to help promote numeracy in health care. http://www.snap.nhs.uk

---

When sitting down to undertake the assessment take note of the following:
- How many questions are on the paper so you complete all of them?
- Be aware of the time allowed to provide your answers.
- Ensure that you include the correct units for all answers where appropriate. Answers will be deemed incorrect if the wrong units are indicated, or if units are not included when they are required.
- You may not be able to use a calculator.
- In some organisations the pass mark is 100%.

The interview

So far so good. Now that your application has been put in the right pile, 'invite for interview', you should be feeling a little more confident. There are a few more hurdles to get over first and of course the biggest one is getting through the interview stage and all that it entails.

In an increasingly highly competitive nursing job market, you want to have an interview that will make a positive and long-lasting impact on the interviewer but, you have to put much effort into this aspect of the job-seeking process.

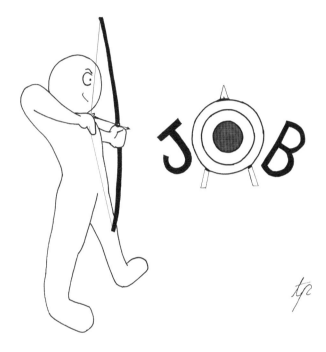

During the interview there are two things you should aim to accomplish:
1 Decide if the organisation is an organisation you want to work for.
2 Convince the interview panel you are the person they want to take on.

The interviewer believes you can do this job, otherwise you would not have come so far in the process; knowing this should boost your confidence.

When you are being interviewed for a nursing position, you will be asked about your skills and your experience, your nurse education programme and your interests. There are a myriad of questions you could be asked. Usually, there are three basic concerns that the interviewing panel will have:
1 What you can do for them
2 Why it is you want to work with them
3 What you are like once they get to know you.

Things to consider

Here are some questions that you might be asked during an interview for a staff nurse's post.

- What made you choose nursing as a career?
- How has your nurse education programme prepared you for the post you are applying for?
- What interests you about working in this trust (organisation)?
- Do you have any professional affiliations?
- What do you do to keep current with regard to nursing and medical practices?
- How do you manage stress?
- How would you manage a situation where a patient or his or her relative wants to make a complaint about your nursing care?
- How would you care for a patient who constantly complains about pain?
- What do you feel you contribute to your patient's health and wellbeing?
- What do you find difficult about being a nurse?
- What do you find are the most rewarding aspects about being a nurse?
- Do you prefer to work alone, or as part of a team?

While the interview panel have questions they want to ask you, you should also prepare your own interview questions. This is not an interrogation, and should be seen as a two-way conversation with both parties having similar agendas. Table 1.6 outlines some of the typical questions that you might wish to ask at interview.

Practicalities

When the invitation to attend interview arrives be sure you know where the interview is to take place, what time and if possible who will be sitting on the panel. Ask if there are any special items you should bring along to the interview. If you are not familiar with the venue where the interview is to take place it is advisable that you make a test run a few days prior to the interview. Even if you know the area you should ask for an informal visit. On the day of interview

Table 1.6 Some questions that you may wish to ask at interview.

- Please describe what you see as a typical day on the job
- Is there room for advancement (caution here: you do not want to appear too pushy)
- Who do you see as the ideal candidate for this position
- To whom would I be reporting
- What continuing professional development opportunities are available
- How will my performance be evaluated and how often
- Please tell me about the overall organisational structure

bring a photocopy of the application form you have completed and your CV in case you need to refer to it during the interview.

Remember the basics, be sure to get a good night's sleep the day before the event and be sure you have had something to eat before the interview. Arrive early for the event – there are no excuses for arriving late for the interview; however, if there is an emergency then let the interviewer know the situation – they may be prepared to wait until you arrive or they may reschedule.

You will need to provide evidence of registration with the NMC; if this is pending then your University will be able to provide you with conformation to say that your registration is currently being processed.

Things to consider

Hints and tips

- Be wise and make allies of everyone along the way – the receptionist, the personal assistant, the secretary.
- Take a pen and pad to make notes during or immediately after the interview.
- While waiting to be called read organisational material or a nursing journal.
- Do not speak negatively of your University during interview.
- If practical, shake hands with each member of the panel and look them in the eye – engage with them.
- Come across as enthusiastic and interested.
- Do not chew gum or smoke.
- Relax.
- Use the interviewer's name from time to time during the interview.
- Use good diction – say 'yes' as opposed to 'yeah'.
- Use active verbs when you talk about your skills and expertise, for example, 'I assessed a patient', 'I instigated a University club', 'I led on a service improvement initiative'.
- Avoid saying 'I think', 'I suppose', 'I guess' – these words can make you come across as less assertive.
- When talking about your skills use positive strong words, avoiding words such as 'pretty well', 'fairly good'.
- Do not apologise for your lack of experience; instead make clear your willingness to remain a lifelong learner and your desire to implement what you have learnt on your programme of study.

It is usual for interviews to be made up of three components:

1 Establishing rapport
2 Exchanging information
3 Closing the interview.

Understanding these three stages will help you. Table 1.7 outlines the anatomy of an interview, the structure of the interview.

Table 1.7 The interview structure.

Establishing rapport	During this stage the interviewer and the interviewee get to know each other; there is some small talk and this will last for about 5 minutes
	Even though this is a relatively short period of time it is an important period – first impressions are important. You should aim to appear confident and competent. Remember it is not only what you say but also what you are doing (your body language); fidgeting can demonstrate anxiety and yawning will demonstrate disinterest
	Sit up straight, looking at the interviewer and learning inwards; this will depict you as an active listener
Exchanging information	This stage is the longest stage of the interview and can last up to 30 minutes. During this stage you will be asked a series of job-related questions
	The interviewer will do the leading here
	Listen carefully to the questions being asked and think about the responses you are going to make
	Again, your posture and body language will be speaking volumes, so be aware of this
	Your aim is to demonstrate that you are motivated and that you want this job, you are interested and you are capable of doing the job. You should be promoting yourself, your traits and how these match the job description
Closing the interview	During this stage the aim is to pull all of the loose ends together
	At this stage you have the opportunity to ask your questions
	If summary questions are being asked then use this opportunity to emphasise your strengths as well as your interest in the position
	Next steps are outlined and if they are not you should ask for clarification on how the process is to proceed
	If you have enjoyed the conversation tell the interviewer this

What to wear for interview

Some people make this their biggest concern; it is, however, a very common question. Typically, nursing candidates should wear professional attire – for men a shirt and tie with trousers, and for women dress pants (or a tailored skirt) and a blouse.

Whatever you decide to wear, be sure that you appear neat and well groomed. Clothes should be pressed, tailored and where possible in neutral colours with a simple or traditional design. Keep accessories to a minimum as well and avoid wearing nail varnish and nail extensions.

Applying for a position overseas

Not all newly qualified nurses stay in the United Kingdom for their first nursing post; some travel overseas to destinations such as Australia, Canada and the Middle East. This work may be paid work or voluntary/humanitarian. There are specific nursing agencies that focus on helping nurses to secure employment abroad.

The RCN has produced a number of resources to assist nurses who wish to seek employment abroad. The resources cover issues such as personal safety, working visa requirements, insurance, immunisations, contract of employment, interviews and job offers.

Conclusion

The day you start your first staff nurse's job will be the first day of the rest of your professional life as a lifelong learner. The last few weeks at University and the transition into your new role as staff nurse can be fraught with a variety of mixed emotions from elation to dread.

Looking for a job can be a challenge; it is no longer an expectation that upon completion of a programme of study leading to registration this will automatically lead to a guaranteed job. There are a limited number of jobs available in some areas for newly qualified nurses; competition can be ferocious and unemployment for some is a real possibility. With perseverance, energy and the right attitude you can get the job that you want but you have to put effort into your endeavours. Preparing for the whole selection process is essential if you are to be successful.

The rest of your professional life is ahead of you and it can be said that learning does not really begin until you leave University and truly embark on your lifelong learning trajectory. All of that learning that has taken place while at University and on your clinical placements will come flooding back once you are in your new role in your new uniform with your new name badge that says staff nurse. Making the changeover from student to staff nurse can be a positive one because you are in the driving seat.

In order to feel competent and comfortable in the new role of staff nurse you will need to be supported. All newly qualified nurses should have access to preceptorship programmes, which will help your mentors help you settle in (DH, 2010) enabling you to become familiar with the environment, staff, patients, role and responsibilities.

References

Department of Health (2010) "Preceptorship Framework for Newly Registered Nurses, Midwives and Allied Healthcare Professionals". DH: London.

Royal College of Nursing (2003) "Defining Nursing" www.rcn.org.uk/publications last (accessed December 2013).

Royal College of Nursing (2005) "Tips for Competing Application Forms and CVs" http://www.rcn.org.uk/_data/assets/pdf_file/0006/264264/Tips_for_completing_application_forms_and_CVs.pdf last (accessed December 2013).

Royal College of Nursing (2013) "The Nursing Team: Common Goals, Different Roles". RCN: London.

Skills for Health (2010) (2nd Ed) "Key Elements of the Career Framework" http://www.skillsforhealth.org.uk/images/stories/Resource-Library/PDF/Career_framework_key_elements.pdf last (accessed December 2013).

Tremayne, V. (2009) "How to Read a Job Advertisement". Nursing Standard, Vol 24, No **12**, pp. 62

CHAPTER 2

Crossing the threshold: the role and function of the staff nurse

Aim

The aim of this chapter is to encourage you to think about your new role in a positive and meaningful manner.

Objectives

By the end of this chapter you will be able to:
1 Understand the issues to be considered when transitioning from student nurse to registered nurse
2 Reflect on the challenges that the staff nurse may face when taking up their first post
3 Outline the role and function of the staff nurse
4 Consider various job descriptions and person specifications
5 Devise methods to address issues that may arise

Introduction

It takes a remarkable person to be a nurse. You will already know what is required of you in your new job as you have now been employed as a staff nurse, hopefully in the job that you really want. The role and function of the registered nurse is complex and often, despite what it says in the job description, the work that you do cannot be reduced to words on a sheet of paper.

The Essential Guide to Becoming a Staff Nurse, First Edition. Ian Peate.
© 2016 John Wiley & Sons, Ltd. Published 2016 by John Wiley & Sons, Ltd.

The transition

The transition from being a student to becoming a staff nurse is a common rite of passage that takes you from the end of your pre-registration undergraduate educational preparation to the beginning of your professional journey as a registered nurse; it is the beginning of your lifelong learning journey – many may say this is the first day of the rest of your life.

There has been much debate over the years concerning the competence of newly qualified staff nurses at the point of registration. You should be proud of your achievements. You have been deemed competent by the educational institution where you studied; the other nurses and health and social care staff who have assessed you in the various learning placements and the Nursing and Midwifery Council have all deemed you competent. What you might lack at this moment in time is confidence but you do not lack competence. The Willis Commission on Nursing Education (Royal College of Nursing – RCN, 2012) has gathered evidence concerning the best methods of delivering pre-registration nursing education in the United Kingdom and how effective the current education system is; the commission considered in particular the balance between workplace and classroom learning. Lord Willis' report concluded that there were no shortcomings in nursing education that could be directly responsible for poor standards of care or a decline in care standards. Furthermore, there was no evidence that degree-level registration was damaging to patient care – nurses are not 'too posh to wash' or 'too clever to care'.

Things to consider

Try not to forget the reasons why you came into nursing. Do not devalue those skills that are so fundamental to the role and function of the registered nurse such as, washing, feeding and helping people to meet their elimination needs.

The transition from student to staff nurse can feel massive and at the same time the fact that you have developed the skills, knowledge and attitude to make a difference is thrilling. However, now there is a difference in expectations, responsibility and above all accountability (Nursing and Midwifery Council, 2015). This transition brings with it the potential to do good but also to do harm, particularly if you are unprepared. This transition is the same for those students who then become registered nurses the world over (Whitehead, 2011) so you are definitely not alone!

Starting a new nursing job is a time filled with promise and expectations, but it is also tinged with uncertainty. You need to let go and welcome new beginnings.

Things to consider

Starting off on the right foot

1 **Take advantage of your position** People will know you are newly qualified so take advantage of each learning opportunity that comes along.

2 **Use your mentor to the maximum** Take every opportunity to work closely with your mentor or preceptor, share in her or his wisdom.

3 **Avoid the 'office politics'** Try not to get caught up in unhealthy dynamics in order to try to fit in. Take a step back, assess the situation and develop an appropriate professional stance.

4 **Become a team member** Build good working relationships with colleagues, offering to help them when they are in a difficult situation. Socialisation is important.

5 **Be open and receptive** Be teachable, open and receptive – do not be afraid to ask questions. Asking questions can also prevent mistakes from happening and misunderstandings occurring.

6 **Be observant** Observe the expert practitioners you are working with – you can learn a lot by watching a good role model at work. Observe how they make decisions, negotiate, handle difficult situations and interact with other members of the multidisciplinary team. Make your own mind up about what works and what does not.

7 **Formulate goals and set priorities** Develop the ability to set short-term and long-term personal and professional goals concerning your future aspirations. Evaluate situations and in so doing this will also enable you to prioritise when working with patients.

8 **Develop networks** Make friends within your own organisation and also externally. Interact with others (service providers such as housekeepers, maintenance staff, other nurses, members of the multidisciplinary team). Interacting with others and developing networks widens your human and physical resources and keeps you abreast of contemporary practice.

9 **Be kind to yourself** Remember to recharge your batteries often. Be aware of your body (mentally and physically) and what it is saying to you – take time to destress (however this is). Looking after yourself will help you look after people more effectively, making you a better nurse. Be easy on yourself.

10 **Give it a chance** Give your new position a chance. For sure there will be times when you become frustrated or discouraged – you will be asking 'what is the point', 'have I made the right decision'; do not give up on yourself or the organisation. Any change is frightening; you should give yourself time to adapt to your new role as a professional. It can take around 6 months to a year to feel that you are fully integrated and part of a team.

The bitter sweet – reality shock

Students, as a result of their status, are viewed as learners and as individuals who require supervision and guidance. After the student has graduated and has had his or her name entered on to the professional register it is at this stage that those protective barriers provided by the educational system disappear and the newly

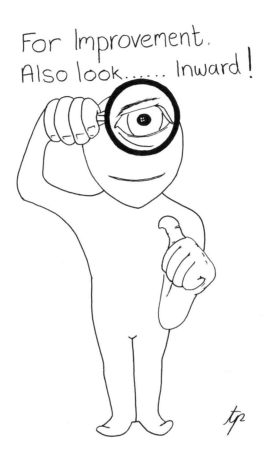

qualified nurse realises that expectations and responsibilities have increased dramatically and with that comes the bitter sweet experience of being a staff nurse.

In 1974 Kramer wrote about 'reality shock', where she described the experience of newly qualified nurses during their first few months of practice – the first 6 months following graduation are acutely stressful for new staff nurses. The reality shock along with its accompanying strain can cause some new nurses to question their abilities, doubt the choice of career, provoke self-doubt; some may even leave the profession. As the novice nurse progresses through the various stages identified by Kramer (1974), role conflict begins to resolve. Over 40 years later, the same theme still applies.

> **Over to you staff nurse**
>
> Think about some of the reasons why nurses leave nursing. Now, consider your reasons with the reasons that Kramer (1974) cites; have things changed much?

The transition from student to practicing nurse varies from person to person. Newly qualified nurses can employ a number of strategies that can help them cope with the shock of reality.

To get through those first difficult months, supportive friends and colleagues are essential; they will answer your questions and show you how to work clinically, undertaking procedures you may not have encountered before. Most newly qualified nurses say they could have done with gaining more clinical experience as a student but, the programme of study is for 3 years only.

Coping strategies vary and often are unique to one person, but there are some general strategies that can be employed to ease the transition from student to nurse. One essential tactic is to find a mentor, someone who can help when the going gets tough and someone who can share your achievements and successes with, no matter how small these may seem. Never regret not reaching out and getting the help you need and remember you are never alone; you can call on a number of people, for example, a nurse lecturer who has taught you, an allocated preceptor or other nurses. Often the best mentors are those who recollect what it was like to be a newly qualified nurse. It is also helpful to be around other newly qualified nurses with whom you can share your anxieties and this will help you not to feel as if you are the only one trying to adjust to new ways, a new role and new experiences (and in some instances a new work environment). Having the opportunity to let off steam with someone who understands and is in the same situation can be an asset.

One of the most important strategies for newly qualified nurses is knowing how to take care of yourself. For you to take care of people effectively, competently, confidently and compassionately you must first learn to take care of yourself, your physical, mental and emotional well-being. Self-care strategies are important and uniquely based on the needs of each individual. Being able to step back and reflect on incidents and issues may help you to make sense of them in a more meaningful manner and to learn from them. Setting boundaries and knowing your limitations and when to ask for, or when to seek help, is not only safe for you but also for the people and families who you offer care to.

It is not possible for the nursing curriculum that you have just engaged with to fully prepare you for that first day on the job as a staff nurse. Whilst university can provide you with the theory underpinning practice, preparing you for your first day is a very different matter; sadly, not everything goes by the textbook.

Soon, however, all the pieces of the puzzle will fit together; the picture becomes clearer and day by day it gets a little easier as your confidence and competence grows helping you to put into practice what you have learnt. Work can be exciting, hectic and rewarding but as is the case with every new nurse, you need to learn about so many things such as time management and how to prioritise. Learning all of these things, how to prioritise, how to manage patients and how to juggle competing demands, how to get along with colleagues just takes time and with time comes experience.

What you do as a nurse matters; it may not be a high-paying job, but what you do really does make a difference to individuals, their families and communities. Being a nurse brings with it challenging and rewarding opportunities to make a positive impact on the lives of people and these people very often are the most vulnerable in our society.

Newly qualified nurses begin their first post with a range of different skills, knowledge and interests; some of these nurses will conquer any deficits they may have and develop more quickly than others. As individuals, they will also have a number of developmental needs that will vary according to the care area in which they are working. It is essential, therefore, for each newly qualified nurse that individual needs are assessed and the emerging differences taken into account when planning development programmes such as preceptorship (see Chapter 3).

Nursing and the NHS

The NHS employed 146,087 doctors, 371,777 qualified nursing staff and 36,360 managers in 2013. There were 23,531 more NHS nurses in 2013 compared to 10 years earlier. The total number, however, has declined in each of the previous 3 years. A total of 2166 more practice nurses were employed by GPs in 2013 than 10 years earlier. Over half of NHS employees are professionally qualified clinical staff. There were 13,974 more qualified allied health professionals and 3968 more health scientists employed in the NHS in 2013 compared to 2003. However, the number within the latter group has declined for each of the past 4 years. Since 2003 the number of professionally qualified clinical staff in the NHS increased by 16.1%. This rise includes an increase in doctors of 34.4%, an increase in the number of nurses of 6.8% along with 17.4% more qualified ambulance staff (NHS Confederation, 2014).

Nursing does not only take place in the NHS; although the NHS is the biggest employer of nurses in the United Kingdom there are other employers that employ nurses to carry out a range of duties. More and more nurses are now working across the health and social care sectors; the intention of the government is to bring these two sectors closer together, and nurses are the catalyst for this to happen.

Nursing careers

Most countries of the United Kingdom are experiencing some of the largest organisational changes to the NHS that have ever been seen since its inception. The challenges faced require reconsideration and a redesign of current systems. The skills and competencies of those working in the health and social care systems (allied health care professionals, community nurses, primary care practitioners and others) should be harnessed in order to meet the needs of patients and their families.

The implementation of the Health and Social Care Act 2012 has brought with it a number of changes that aim to safeguard the NHS and to change the way it functions in order to meet the challenges it will face in the future and to avoid problems that may be encountered tomorrow. By bringing together a number of services in health and social care (the integration of services) it is anticipated that this will offer a seamless patient journey, ensuring that the patient is at the heart of all that we do. In order for these aspirations to become a reality nurses are required to change the way that they work and function; this brings with it opportunity and challenge.

It must be remembered, however, that nurses do not work in isolation and the nursing team consists of more than registered nurses. As nursing careers are being modernised so too are the careers of other professional groups. This must be taken into account when the role of the nurse is being reconfigured in order to take into account the profound changes that are taking place with regard to the way health and social care is being delivered. The key aim has to be to ensure that any modernisation of nursing careers is flexible, diverse and rewarding and that patients receive a high-quality service provided by nurses who are confident in what they do.

Modernising nursing careers

In 2006 the four Chief Nursing Officers of the United Kingdom met to consider the ways in which the careers of nurses could be modernised in response to and in step with the changing needs of the people of the United Kingdom as well as the career aspirations of nurses.

Over to you staff nurse

Explore the different career opportunities that are available, think about them in the short term and the long term and discuss these options with colleagues – what do you need to start thinking about now, what goals should you be setting in order to be more prepared when these opportunities become available.

There were four key recommendations arising from the work of the four Chief Nursing Officers (DH, 2006):

1 Develop a competent and flexible nursing workforce
2 Update career pathways and career choices
3 Prepare nurses to lead in a changed health care system
4 Modernise the image of nursing and nursing careers.

The Health Departments worked with stakeholders in order to agree and communicate key messages concerning nursing and nursing careers; one aspect of this was to provide information for the public on what it is that nurses actually do – the aim was to address the outdated image of the nurse often based on media stereotypes.

Other health policy drivers underpinned this work and these included:

• More health and nursing care to be delivered in the community setting
• Increasing e-technology and informatics in the delivery of health care
• Acute hospital inpatient care to move towards more short stay and critical care interventions
• The growing number of health care providers, such as, social enterprise models
• The need to focus more in the future on the management of chronic and long-term conditions and public health.

Table 2.1 provides an overview of the direction that the DH (2006) wished the future of nursing careers to take.

Over to you staff nurse

Consider the content of table 2.1 and identify those areas where there have been developments in the aspirations of the Chief Nursing Officers.

Table 2.1 Modernising nursing careers.

Coming from	Going towards
Outdated image of nursing careers dictated by media stereotypes	An up-to-date picture of nursing careers characterised by opportunity and diversity
A nursing workforce focused on hospital-based care	Care taking place in and outside hospital with the workforce moving between. Nurses starting their career in the community
One point of entry to nursing	A career framework allowing nursing to 'grow its own' with multiple entry points for those taking up nursing as a second career or as mature entrants
Working for the NHS as the only employer	Plurality of provision offering alternative employers and employment models including NHS Foundation Trusts, self-employment and social enterprises
An education system with a one-size-fits-all approach, struggling to balance academic and practical learning and reflective of health care today, not tomorrow	A flexible principle-based curriculum that is built around patient pathways, with a strong academic foundation and interdisciplinary learning
Linear careers based on increasing specialisation or promotion out of practice, with consequences for those stepping off or changing pathway	A framework that supports movement between career pathways, practice, management and education, and that values and rewards different career types
Increasing specialisation and sub-specialisation	Better balance of generalists and specialists to provide integrated networks of urgent, specialist and continuing care
Careers described by discipline or setting	Careers built around patient pathways using competence as the currency for greater movement and flexibility
Career structure with few opportunities for assistants	A career structure with increased number of assistants working as part of multidisciplinary teams

(continued overleaf)

Table 2.1 (*continued*)

Coming from		Going towards
No standardisation of advanced-level skills	→	Standardisation of advanced-level skills
Organisation-based careers with an abundance of titles	→	Patient pathway-based careers focusing on nursing roles rather than titles
Role based on title	→	Nursing roles defined according to patient need to provide intervention that is timely, accurate and swift
Nursing teams managed hierarchically	→	Nursing teams more self-directed and professionally accountable
Nurses involved mainly in giving care	→	Nurses leading, coordinating and commissioning care, as well as giving care, to bring about change measured by health gain and health outcomes
Care influenced by custom and practice	→	Care based on evidence and critical thinking and assisted by new technology

Source: Adapted from Department of Health (2004).

Nursing careers framework

There are a number of competencies required that nurses have to meet in order to step onto a 'career framework'. Figure 2.1 is an adaptation of the key elements of the careers framework that is used by Skills for Health (2010). The framework is composed of nine different levels at which various functions could be performed, beginning at level 1 roles to more senior levels for more senior staff at level 9.

Over to you staff nurse

Go to figure 2.1 and make an assessment of where you are now in your career trajectory and then consider what you wish to aspire to in the future.

See if you can obtain copies of job descriptions for those who work at career framework levels 8 and 9 and map the job description across to the elements listed in the framework.

9 **Career framework level 9**
People working at level 9 require knowledge at the most advanced frontier of the field of work and at the interface between fields. They will have responsibility for the development and delivery of a service to a population, at the highest level of the organisation. **Indicative or Reference title: Director**

8 **Career framework level 8**
Nurses at level 8 require highly specialised knowledge, some of which is at the forefront of knowledge in a field of work, they use this as the basis for original thinking and/or research. They are leaders with considerable responsibility, researching and analysing complex processes. They have responsibility for service improvement or development. They may have significant clinical and/or management responsibilities, are accountable for service delivery or have a leading education or commissioning role. **Title: Consultant/Expert Nurse**

7 **Career framework level 7**
Those at level 7 have a critical awareness of knowledge, issues in the field and also with other fields. These nurses are innovative, have a responsibility for developing and changing practice and/or services in a complex and unpredictable environment. **Title: Advanced Practitioner**

6 **Career framework level 6**
People at level 6 must have a critical understanding of detailed theoretical and practical knowledge, are specialists and/or have management and leadership responsibilities. They use initiative and are creative when finding solutions to problems. They have some responsibility for team performance and service development, undertaking self development. **Title: Specialist/Senior Practitioner**

5 **Career framework level 5**
Nurses at this level have a comprehensive, specialised, factual and theoretical knowledge within a field of work, they are aware of their boundaries. They use knowledge to solve problems creatively, make judgements which require analysis and interpretation, and actively contribute to service and self development. They can have responsibility for supervision of staff. **Title: Practitioner**

4 **Career framework level 4**
People at career framework level 4 require factual and theoretical knowledge in broad contexts within a field of work. They are guided by standard operating procedures, protocols or systems of work, they make judgements, plan activities, contribute to service development and demonstrate self development. They may have responsibility for supervision of some staff. **Title: Assistant/Associate Practitioner**

3 **Career framework level 3**
Nurses at level 3 require knowledge of facts, principles, processes and general concepts in a field of work. They carry out a wider range of duties than those working at level 2, and have more responsibility, with guidance and supervision available when required. They contribute to service development, and are responsible for self development. **Title: Senior Healthcare Assistant/Technician**

2 **Career framework level 2**
People at level 2 require basic factual knowledge of a field of work. They carry out clinical, technical, scientific or administrative duties adhering to established protocols or procedures, or systems or work. **Title: Health Care Assistant/Support Worker**

1 **Career framework level 1**
Those at level 1 are at entry level, requiring basic general knowledge, undertaking a limited number of basic tasks under direct supervision. **Title: Health Care Assistant/Cadet**

Figure 2.1 Key elements of the career framework. Source: Adapted from Skills for Health 2010) and Benner (1984).

Not all employers use this framework but it will give you an idea of where you are now and what you can aspire to in the future. Local career frameworks are often developed to meet local organisational needs.

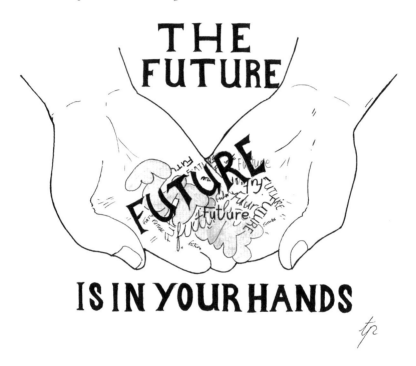

Health and society

The NHS Confederation (2014) note that life expectancy for men in 2008–2010 was 78.2 years and that for women 82.3 years in the United Kingdom. The population is expected to increase from a projected 62.26 million in 2010 to 71.39 million by 2030. The number of people aged 65 years and above is destined to grow to 15,778,000 by 2031. It has been estimated that there are over 2.8 million people with diabetes in the United Kingdom; this is double the number from 1996 and by 2025 is predicted to reach 4 million. The proportion of men in the United Kingdom who have been classified as obese increased from 13.2% in 1993 to 26.2% in 2010 and for women from 16.4% to 26.1% over the same timescale.

These changes in health and population are having and will have a significant impact on the role and function of the nurse. Nursing roles must develop to meet

Table 2.2 Trends interrelated with health and society.

- Rapid and ongoing changes in technology and patient education
- Significant societal demographic changes
- The economy and consequences of the economy crisis
- Globalisation of knowledge and disease
- Increasing demands being made on health care provider's competence
- Complexity of physical and mental health conditions
- Impact of ethical issues
- Shortage of nursing and other health care professionals
- Changes to nurse education
- Changes in consumer demand and expectation
- Changes in statutory and voluntary provision
- Health and social care reform

the needs of the population and as the population demography changes so too does the way in which health and social services are delivered. Society as a whole is going through many significant changes and these will influence how the art and science of nursing is carried out.

The role of the nurse has changed significantly but not beyond recognition. Nursing is becoming more complex and the role as a registered nurse is more demanding and this requires you to become more involved in high-level care decisions. Nurses must be effective and efficient in understanding how societal and health care changes can impact on health outcomes.

Society in the United Kingdom is becoming more diverse and complex with new trends precipitating a variety of issues. Competent and confident nurses integrate these changes into their way of being and they become thinking as well as doing nurses, ensuing that the patient is at the centre of all they do. Integration of knowledge, skills and attitudes is essential along with practice that is underpinned by an evidence base in order to promote patient safety and to offer high-quality care. Table 2.2 outlines some of the issues that are associated with health and society.

The role

When carrying out your role you have the potential to affect every person (and families) that you meet. Nurses help people to live lives that are healthier, and offer support to those with a disability or to those who have chronic disorders with the intention of helping them achieve their full potential. Caring for people with a terminal illness and helping them experience a dignified death are also central activities associated with the complex role of the nurse. As you know, no two 24 hours in nursing will ever be the same and no two patients you meet will be the same either.

We all have preferences about the nature and type of work we enjoy. As you make the transition through your first year as a newly registered nurse you will have experiences which will shape and inform your future career choices. The experiences you have had as a student nurse may well have led you to the job where you are today.

The Career Framework for Health and the NHS Knowledge and Skills Framework

Nurses across the United Kingdom hold the same core values regardless of the country in which they work. Nurses want a vibrant and flexible career structure and they welcome opportunities to expand and develop their roles and capabilities. Career development is important for individual nurses, employers and most importantly patients, as well as their carers. Career progression is not always about promotion to a higher grade, which may bring with it a higher salary; it is often about personal and professional development expanding knowledge, skills and altitudes from a competent level to an advanced practitioner and expert level.

The Career Framework for Health and the NHS Knowledge and Skills Framework (NHS KSF) (DH, 2004) was a tool that was developed to support career and pay progression within the Agenda for Change pay scheme in the NHS; the NHS KSF is applicable to all staff with the exception of doctors and dentists. The KSF provides definitions and offers descriptions of the knowledge and skills that staff employed in the NHS will apply in their work with the aim of delivering safe and quality services. It was produced to provide a single, consistent, comprehensive and clear framework on which to base review and development for all NHS staff. The KSF has an organising structure of dimensions and levels under which is more detail of performance indicators and spheres of application. Organisations then apply this overall framework to the roles and jobs in that organisation. The KSF is broad and generic in nature as a result of the 1 million plus NHS staff it is required to cover. The Royal College of Nursing, UNISON and UNITE provide additional detail that can be used to show how nurses meet the requirements of the NHS KSF (see e.g. RCN, 2009). It is important to understand the fundamental elements of the KSF as this may impact on career and pay progression within the service.

The NHS KSF focuses on a range of dimensions. There are six core dimensions; these cover the key areas that are applicable to every job. They contain examples of behaviours and actions that will support appraisal discussions and help

Table 2.3 The six core dimensions that
are applicable to all NHS posts.

1 Communication
2 Personal and people development
3 Health, safety and security
4 Service improvement
5 Quality
6 Equality and diversity

Source: Department of Health (2004). Reproduced with permission of Crown Copyright.

Over to you staff nurse

Find the pay scales for the following nursing positions:
- Consultant nurse
- Clinical nurse specialist
- Charge nurse
- Senior staff nurse.

How easy was it to do that? Did you struggle with job titles? Might it
have been easier to complete the action point had you been asked to consider bands as opposed to job titles?

---

determine if a particular dimension is being met or not. Table 2.3 provides a list
of the six dimensions.

As well as the core dimensions there are also specific dimensions that are
related to specific aspects of the nurses' role and level that is appropriate for the
post. There are 24 specific dimensions grouped in four categories. Each dimension is divided into four levels – the higher the level the greater the level of
expectations of knowledge and skill for the post (RCN, 2007). Most posts will
have no more than a maximum of seven additional dimensions. Table 2.4 provides a list of these specific dimensions.

The job description

Job descriptions are statements that provide you with an overview of:
- Duties
- Responsibilities
- Key contributions and outcomes needed from the position
- Necessary qualifications of candidates
- Reporting relationship of a particular job.

Table 2.4 Specific dimensions.

1 Health and well-being (HWB)
2 Estates and facilities (EI)*
3 Information and knowledge (IK)
4 General (G)

*The specific dimension estates and facilities is not applicable to any nursing post at any level.

Job descriptions are based on objective information that is obtained through job analysis, an understanding of the competencies and skills required to accomplish needed tasks and the needs of the organisation to produce work; they also take into account the NHS KSFs.

There are generic elements of a job description as well as specific aspects; for example, a staff nurse's post in a dementia unit will have generic aspects such as communication and relationship skills, responsibility for assessing, planning, implementing and evaluating care as will a staff nurse's post in a medical investigations unit. Table 2.5 provides information concerning the elements of a band 5 staff nurse's job profile; most of these elements would be present in a band 5 staff nurse's job description.

The job description along with the job profile and the NHS KSFs attempt to spell out the responsibilities of a specific job. Table 2.5 includes information about working conditions, tools, equipment used, knowledge and skills needed and relationships with other people.

Things to consider

There are high-level skills associated with the delegation and assigning of tasks to others. Supervision of those to whom you have delegated a task or duty is an essential competency for all registered nurses working in all health care settings. Any decisions you make concerning delegation must be based on the principles of safety and your concern for protecting the public.

Job descriptions do and should change they are updated as responsibilities change. They do not limit the employee, but instead, can let them stretch their experience, develop skills and enhance their ability to contribute to the work and overall aims of the organisation.

Over to you staff nurse

When nurses are considering which tasks and activities to delegate to others what should you be considering and why?

Table 2.5 Aspects of job profile that are related to the work of a band 5 staff nurse.

Elements of the role	Description
Commutation and relationship skills	Provides and receives complex, sensitive information
Knowledge, training and experience	Applies professional expertise and clinical knowledge acquired through training
Analytical and judgement skills	Applies judgement on problems such as the analysis of assessment data related to a person's condition
Planning and organisational skills	Organises own time and the time of others such as junior staff and students
Physical skills	Requires dexterity and accuracy in order to provide care and work with equipment
Responsibility for policy/service development	Adheres to policy and procedures and is professionally accountable
Responsibility for physical and financial resources	Has a personal duty of care with regard to equipment and resources; handles cash and patient valuables
Responsibility for the use of human resources	Supervises other junior staff and students; is professionally accountable for any work delegated
Responsibility for information resources	Maintains patient records
Responsibility for research and development	Undertakes or participates in research and development activity
Freedom to act	Works within the auspices of codes of conduct and adheres to professional guidance
Physical exertion	Is required to undertake physical activity that can involve sitting, standing, pushing/pulling/manoeuvring patients
Mental exertion	Is required to concentrate for a number of purposes, for example, the calculation of drug dosages
Emotional exertion	Cares for distressed patients, relatives, people who are terminally ill, death and dying
Working conditions	Exposed to unpleasant smells and sights; deals with body fluids

Developing your role

The nursing role is rapidly evolving as nurses take on an even wider range of health care responsibilities. Caring for the sick and preventing illness has become more complicated. Financial constraints are impacting on all aspects of health care and in particular with regard to staffing – budgets are tight.

Political and regulatory landscapes are constantly changing and what they might look like in the future is unclear. Health care reform has and will continue to reshape the nursing profession. In clinics, hospitals and care centres around the United Kingdom, nurses are rising to meet these challenges; progressive nursing education is empowering nurses to lead the way.

The role of the nurse is much more than caring for the sick; nurses are changing the very concept of modern health care delivery and are actively addressing and formulating health care policy. The field is growing and along with this also comes numerous openings for nurses and nursing.

Things to consider

Career goals

Lawton and Wimpenny (2003) suggest that one of the most important skills for managing a successful career is goal setting. The following frameworks may help you set goals that are realistic and effective.

Be wise:

W Workable – based in the reality of the workplace
I Intelligent – thorough and takes into account a wide range of ideas and issues
S Situated – in the group of relationships in the organisation
E Experimental – willing to take risks, experience new ways and generate new aims.

Be open:

O Open – open to a range of ideas and influences
P Participative – stressing inclusivity and mutual learning
E Experiential – seeing learning as situated in reflection on experience
N New knowledge – creating new knowledge as opposed to managing what is known.

Using your preferred framework, think about career goals for the next 2–5 years.

Opportunities for nurses are also coming about as health care technologies advance, for example, mobile devices, electronic medical records and teleconferencing encouraging nurses to become more digitally aware. In the growing field of nursing informatics, nurses are connecting with technology developers to develop systems that are more user friendly. At home monitoring programmes (close to the patient systems), where nurses see patients on live webcasts, are in some parts of the United Kingdom playing a larger role in patient care.

These emerging tools are at the front of more cost-efficient health care delivery and those nurses who can adapt and implement technology will become much sought after. Also evolving in a digitalized world are patient behaviours. More patients are accessing online resources to research and seek treatment of their symptoms. On the search engine Google, health and wellness are constantly among the most searched for topics. Nurses will be required to help patients with regard to the most dependable websites and most useful applications that are available.

It is essential to note that new technologies will not remove the need for traditional care; it will however open up more creative possibilities to offer patient-centred education related to their health. The skilled hands-on experience provided by nurses will be supplemented by the myriad of new technologies. A one-size-fits-all approach to health care provision and patient education is no longer acceptable.

There are hundreds of new medical apps available on the market, from glucose monitors to hypnotic sleep remedies. Offering support to those patients who are thinking of engaging with this type of technology demands that the nurse is knowledgeable or at least able to provide the patient with a contact who can advise them.

Nurses are mastering complex, multifaceted issues that impact the health care system and the health and well-being of the nation. It is more than knowing how to perform tasks and procedures'; nursing is about being a more effective member of the health care team and being able to steer clinical systems in order to respond to a dynamic consumer of health and social care.

Nurses do not only consider the symptoms of patients they meet, they are also required to look at the health of communities and beyond and doing this they have to demonstrate that they are culturally aware. Health care facilities, hospitals and clinics are increasingly diverse where nurses offer care to a multiplicity of people from a variety of ethnic backgrounds, with a diversity of religious beliefs, gender and socioeconomic status.

As nursing becomes more complex there is a need for nurses to be more than competent and confident caregivers; they must also be able to innovate, ensuring that at all times the person being cared for is central to this. Nursing continues to be a profession for those who are intellectually curious and for those who subscribe to the notion of lifelong learner. Regardless of the changes to role and function, at the heart of the profession is the desire to offer care that is safe, effective and delivered with kindness, care and compassion. Nurses are and will remain the caregiver acting as advocate for the most sick and vulnerable of our society.

Effective nurses, nurses who stand out, and nurses who are driven by professional values use what they learn (formally and informally) adapting the key concepts, applying the available evidence, using policy initiatives that are community centred in order to make high level decisions day in and day out.

With the right skills, knowledge and attitude you are now in a position to make a bigger difference to patients, communities and the NHS. The KSF outline is related explicitly to the job description. Your individual development needs will be discussed and are identified through your performance review (sometimes called appraisal or individual performance review (IPR)).

It has to be acknowledged that each person will develop at his or her own speed progressing in different ways bringing with them a number of skills and knowledge. As the nurse and the nurse's career progresses and experience mounts there will be added responsibilities; however, along with this comes that central tenet of professional nursing practice, accountability. Management skills grow, confidence is bolstered and you become much more aware of your projected career pathway; you are moving from competent, to proficient to expert (Benner, 1984). Beware, however, that you do not start to run before you can walk – remember that old adage that pride often comes before a fall; on the other hand, do not be reticent, be confident and assertive in what you do.

Things to consider

A person who is extremely proud of his or her abilities is likely to experience a setback or failure as he or she is inclined to be overconfident and is likely to make errors of judgement. Look before you leap.

Conclusion

The world is your oyster now that you are a registered nurse. You have a licence to practise and that should be seen as a privilege.

Try not to rest on your laurels; in order to remain on the register there are a number of requirements you need to satisfy the Nursing and Midwifery Council with. You will (if not already) be thinking of the future and the direction you want your professional career to go in.

No nurse education programme would ever be able to fully prepare you for the massive transition from student to staff nurse. Much of the success in this transition is down to you, considerable planning and a great deal of good luck. In lots of respect you are now required to change your identity; look at your name badge – it says staff nurse. The title registered nurse is one that is protected in law; use it, you have earned it but respect it also; you are now an autonomous and accountable practitioner. People's expectations of you and your expectations of you have changed; you have to let go now and welcome those new beginnings, build your confidence and develop your understanding.

References

Benner, P. (1984) "From Novice to expert. Excellence and Power in Clinical Nursing Practice". Addison-Wesley: Menlo Park, CA.

Department of Health (2004) "The Knowledge and Skills Framework (NHS KSF) and the Development Review Process". DH: London.

Department of Health (2006) "Modernising Nursing Careers – Setting the Direction". DH: London.

Kramer, M. (1974) "Reality Shock: Why Nurses Leave Nursing". Mosby: St Louis.

Lawton, S. and Wimpenny, P. (2003) "Continuing Professional Development: A Review". Nursing Standard, Vol 17, No **24**, pp. 41–44.

NHS Confederation (2014) "Key Statistics on the NHS" http://www.nhsconfed.org/resources/key-statistics-on-the-nhs last (accessed June 2014).

Nursing and Midwifery Council (2015) "The Code. Professional Standards of Practice and Behaviour for Nurses and Midwives" http://www.nmc-uk.org/Documents/NMC-Publications/NMC-Code-A5-FINAL.pdf last (accessed January 2015).

Royal College of Nursing (2007) "Information for Nursing Students. Outlining the NHS Knowledge and Skills Framework". RCN: London.

Royal College of Nursing (2009) "Integrated Core Career and Competence Framework for Registered Nurses". RCN: London.

Royal College of Nursing (2012) "Quality with Compassion: The Future of Nursing Education. Report of the Willis Commission on Nursing Education" http://www.williscommission.org.uk/__data/assets/pdf_file/0007/495115/Willis_commission_report_Jan_2013.pdf last (accessed June 2014).

Skills for Health (2010) "Key Elements of the Career Framework" http://www.skillsforhealth.org.uk/index.php?option=com_mtree&task=att_download&link_id=163&cf_id=24 last (accessed September 2015).

Whitehead, B. (2011) "Are Newly Qualified Nurse Prepared for Practice?" Nursing Times, Vol 107, No **19–20**, pp. 20–23.

CHAPTER 3

Support systems and preceptorship

Aim

The aim of this chapter is to encourage you to understand the various support systems available to you as you embark on your new career and to value the notion of preceptorship.

Objectives

By the end of this chapter you will be able to:
1. List the various formal and informal support systems available to you
2. Define the concept preceptorship
3. Outline the components of a preceptorship programme
4. Describe the best ways to make use of preceptorship programmes
5. Understand how local induction programmes, mandatory and discretionary training, come together with the intention of developing safe and effective practitioners

Introduction

During your time as a student a number of support systems were put in place to help you navigate, undertake and successfully complete your course of study.

It could be that the first support system you thought about was your peers; you may have also mentioned your family. These systems are just as important now that you are a staff nurse.

The Essential Guide to Becoming a Staff Nurse, First Edition. Ian Peate.
© 2016 John Wiley & Sons, Ltd. Published 2016 by John Wiley & Sons, Ltd.

Universities are required to have in place systems that help students complete their programme of education. They often consider this from an academic and pastoral perspective, offering the following support mechanisms:

- Programme leader
- Module leader
- Personal tutor
- Clinical facilitator
- Occupational health services
- Counselling service
- Services that provide spiritual services (Chaplaincy)
- Access to trade unions such as the Royal College of Nursing, UNISON and UNITE
- National Union of Students.

Over to you staff nurse

Make a list of the support systems that were available to you to help you successfully complete your nurse education programme.

Did you make use of those systems? Did you make enough use of those systems? Were they helpful to you?

Most organisations where you work will provide you with similar services designed to offer you support and also to ensure that you contribute safely and effectively to organisational goals and strategies.

Over to you staff nurse

Now, list the services offered by your employer to help you make a smooth transition from student to staff nurse and beyond.

Preceptorship

The DH (2010) define preceptorship as a period of structured transition for the newly registered nurse during which time he or she will be provided with support by a preceptor, to help and guide him or her develop confidence as an autonomous professional, refine the skills, values and behaviours and to continue on his or her journey of lifelong learning. DeCicco (2008) suggests that preceptorship programmes are used in the health care sector in order to educate nurses, enhance their leadership skills and enrich their quality of work life.

Things to consider

Getting the most out of your period of preceptorship means engaging with the process and ensuring you engage with your preceptor. Remember that the idea is to guide you into full-time work seamlessly. Review your progress on a regular basis.

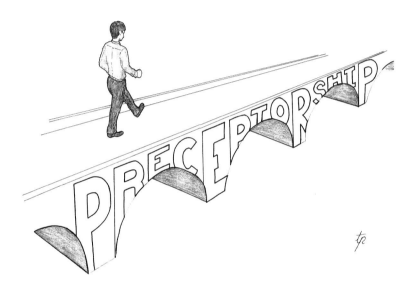

The thinking around preceptorship (the philosophy underpinning it) is to enable newly qualified nurses to consolidate and strengthen their knowledge, to be introduced into the policies and procedures of the workplace and to encourage them to reflect on their practice, particularly with regard to challenging experiences and the change in their role. When the period of preceptorship ends, nurses should feel secure in their role and confident about engaging with regular clinical supervision (continuing professional development) throughout their professional careers, along with, as appropriate, periods of mentorship. The overall aim of the preceptorship phase is to introduce and promote independence and to confirm good clinical practice in a number of situations and settings. Robinson and Griffith (2009) suggest that preceptorship comprises an agreed period of time offering support and guidance for newly qualified

Table 3.1 Three supporting roles.

Preceptor	Coach	Mentor
The preceptor guides the newly qualified nurse into the real world of practice, allowing him or her to try new skills while gaining confidence and validation The preceptor teaches, supports, counsels, coaches, evaluates, serves as a role model and helps the new nurse to socialise into a new role	A coach helps an individual focus on a specific aspect of behaviour, performance or life, focusing on learning and self-awareness, helping the person find his or her own best answers	A mentor looks after and steers the novice through a more personal, long-term relationship. Usually the mentor helps the individual, helping him or her gain entry into places and experiences he or she may not have accessed on his or her own

registrants, allowing them to work competently and independently in their sphere of practice. Table 3.1 offers a distinction between preceptor, coach and mentor.

The DH (2010) consider a newly registered practitioner to be a nurse, midwife or allied health professional who is entering employment in England for the first time following professional registration with the Nursing and Midwifery Council (NMC) or HCPC. It also includes those who are recently graduated students, those who are returning to practice, those entering a new part of the register, for example, community public health specialists and overseas-prepared practitioners who have satisfied the requirements of, and are registered with, the NMC. While participating in preceptorship the newly registered nurse is sometimes known as the 'preceptee'.

Things to consider

Nobody will spoon-feed you on your journey to becoming an expert practitioner. You have to make the effort and your preceptor will expect you to make the first move.

It is expected that the nurse, during the period of preceptorship, will work with his or her preceptor for an explicit period of time during the working week. There is no time limit placed on the period of preceptorship; it is, however, subject to the production and development of a learning contract (an agreement) that sets out mutually agreed goals in relation to decision making and knowledge that

Newly Qualified Registrant (preceptee)
I pledge to assume my responsibilities as a registered practitioner, including to:
- Adhere at all times to the regulatory body requirements for my profession
- Ensure that I understand the standards, competencies or objectives set by my employer that are required to be met
- Commit time to preceptorship
- Work collaboratively with my preceptor to identify, plan and achieve my learning needs
- Take responsibility for my own learning and development
- Provide feedback to enable preceptorship to develop further

Preceptor
I commit to delivering my responsibilities as a preceptor, including to:
- Commit to the preceptorship role and its responsibilities
- Personalise the newly qualified registrant's learning and development needs and help him or her to identify key learning opportunities and resources
- Commit time and provide constructive feedback to support the newly qualified registrant

Signed preceptee_____

Signed preceptor_____

Figure 3.1 A template that can be used as the basis for the preceptee and preceptor agreement.

is steeped in the context of the delivery of safe and effective, evidence-based patient care. Figure 3.1 provides a template that can be used as the basis for the preceptee and preceptor when formulating an agreement.

Over to you staff nurse

Thinking of the content of the agreement (figure 3.1), is there anything else that you would like to add to this agreement?

Preceptorship ends when the preceptor, registered practitioner and manager all agree that the mutual goals set have been achieved. The process has to be incorporated into the staff development activity that is already in place within the organisation and its various departments.

The employer should also enter into an agreement with the preceptor and the 'new registrant', whereby they commit to delivering responsibilities for preceptorship; the following may be a part of that tripartite agreement:

- Ensure that all new registrants have equitable access to preceptorship as well as appropriate access to an identified, suitably prepared preceptor.
- Provide adequate resources for preceptorship.
- Ensure that a system is in place for appraising the preceptee's performance through the NHS Knowledge and Skills Framework or another structure to support appraisal.
- Undertake an evaluation of the process and the outcomes of preceptorship.

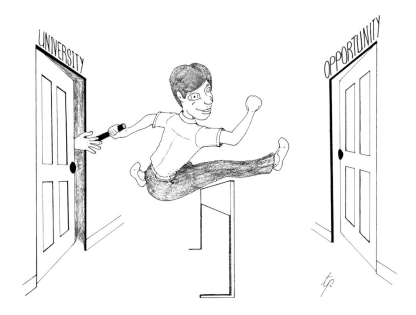

In 2006 the NMC strongly recommended that all newly qualified nurses (and midwives) engage in a period of preceptorship when they commence employment (NMC, 2006). The NMC (2006) considers preceptorship to be about providing support and guidance that will enable 'new registrants' to make the transition from student to accountable practitioner to:

- Practise in association with the NMC's (2015) 'Professional Standards of Practice and Behaviour for Nurses and Midwives'
- Develop confidence in their competence as a nurse.

To enable this to happen the 'new registrant' was is required to have:

- Protected learning time in their first year of qualified practice
- Access to a preceptor with whom regular meetings are held.

> #### Over to you staff nurse
>
> Outline the skills you think a preceptor needs in order to act as an effective preceptor. Does your list match the list below – the preceptor and the role of the preceptor?

The preceptor and the role of the preceptor should be to:
• Facilitate the transition of the 'new registrant' from a student to a registrant who is:
  ◦ confident in her/his practice
  ◦ sensitive to the needs of patients/clients
  ◦ an effective team member
  ◦ up to date with his/her knowledge and practice.
• Offer positive feedback to 'new registrants' on those elements of performance that are being undertaken well.
• Provide honest, appropriate and objective feedback on those aspects of performance that may be a cause for concern and support the 'new registrant' to develop a plan of action to remedy these deficits.
• Facilitate 'new registrants' to gain new knowledge and skills.
• Be aware of the standards, competencies, or objectives set by the employer that the 'new registrant' is to achieve and encourage them in realising these.
• The nature of the relationship between the preceptor and the 'new registrant' is best agreed in accordance with their own needs taking account of the environment within which they practise.

The 'new registrant' has a role to play and the NMC is of the opinion that the 'new registrant' who is receiving preceptorship also has responsibilities; these can be found in table 3.2.

Table 3.2 The expected role of the 'new registrant' in the preceptorship relationship.

• Practise in accordance with the NMC code of professional conduct: standards for conduct, performance and ethics
• Identify and meet with their preceptor as soon as is possible after they have taken up post
• Identify specific learning needs and develop an action plan for addressing these needs
• Ensure that they understand the standard, competencies or objectives set by the employer that they are required to meet
• Reflect on their practice and experience
• Seek feedback on their performance from their preceptor and those with whom they work

---

Source: Adapted from Nursing and Midwifery Council (2006).

Over to you staff nurse

Use this plan (alter it, add to it, delete items from it, make it your own) to help you formulate your own personal development plan and then, if you wish share it with your preceptor.

My greatest strengths are:
1.
2.
3.
4.
5.

My greatest opportunities for improvement are:
1.
2.
3.
4.
5.

How do I plan to improve?

What resources (human and material) will I use?

How will I eliminate any barriers to improvement?

What time frames are appropriate for achieving these plans?

Period of preceptorship

There is no absolute period of time that is allocated to preceptorship, that is, how long it should take to complete. The NMC strongly recommends that all 'new registrants' should have a formal period of preceptorship, around 4 months; however, this may vary according to individual needs as well as local circumstances (NMC, 2006). Preceptorship is contingent upon 'new registrants' having easy access to a named person who is on the same part of the register and the same field of practice, who can provide guidance, help, and offer assistance and support. The NMC's guidelines can be incorporated within current systems and structures for supporting 'new registrants' such as, personal development planning.

It is acknowledged that not all 'new registrants' are employed within large organisations or the NHS. Those who are self-employed or intend to practise intermittently should make arrangements to receive support that meets the principles of the NMC's guidelines.

Preparation for preceptors

In contrast to mentorship, there are no formal qualifications associated with being a preceptor; however, individuals will need to receive preparation for the responsibility. Preceptors should be first level registered nurses who have had at least 12 months experience within the same area of practice as the 'new registrant'. It is expected (but not essential) that those who act as and undertake the role of a preceptor will have undertaken and successfully completed a mentor or practice teacher programme (or equivalent).

Documenting activity

Preceptorship programmes will usually contain formal assessments and it is usual for the preceptees to provide evidence to demonstrate that they have met all the standards in each assessment by the time they reach the end of the programme; these outcomes and standards are usually linked to the NHS Knowledge and Skills Framework. The preceptee is responsible for obtaining the evidence, storing it and reproducing it when needed. The evidence can come from a variety of sources (see figure 3.2).

There are several general principles that underpin the assessment process:

- The assessments are contained within a preceptorship workbook in which evidence is collected and recorded.
- It is expected that the preceptee completes all the formal assessments of the programme and is responsible for maintaining a portfolio of evidence of competence related to specified learning outcomes for each assessment.
- The preceptorship programme documentation reflects the NHS KSF portfolio; the minimum expectation is that all preceptees will complete all the formal assessments specified. More may be added in the form of a development plan if required.
- A named preceptor is identified before the programme begins. The preceptee is required to work with/shadow the preceptor or a nominated deputy for a minimum period of time.
- The preceptor and the preceptee are required to meet for an hour each week for the first month and then monthly for subsequent development meetings until the programme completes. Informal meetings can be held if such a meeting is required. All meetings must be documented.

- The preceptorship process often runs together with any existing staff inductions – this programme does not replace the induction process.
- It is essential that all the assessments are undertaken, even if the preceptee has recently completed any similar assessment (e.g. assessment of drug administration as a student nurse).

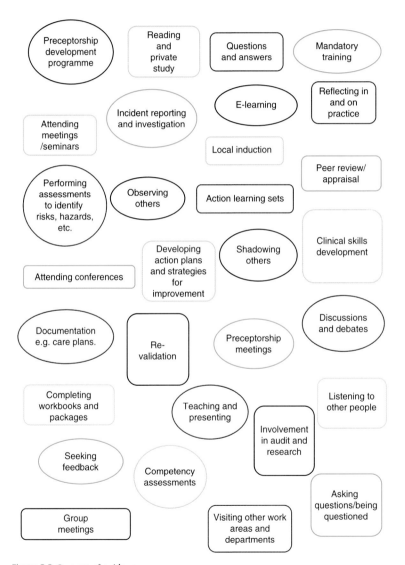

Figure 3.2 Sources of evidence.

Competence

All nurses at the point of registration are competent to practise autonomously in their discipline at the initial level; this is a NMC requirement (NMC, 2010a). Those skills (clinical and otherwise) gained during the nurse's pre-registration period need to be consolidated in order to provide the foundations for continuing development. Registered nurses undertake a broad range of activities in the delivery of care for patients in a number of settings. The nurse is an essential member of the clinical team working to deliver high-quality clinical care.

Accreditation is attained as the nurse will have completed a recognised programme of study as a student that had been validated and accredited by the NMC, which entitles them to apply for their name to be entered on to the professional register.

After registration the nurse is required to undertake post registration continuing professional development (this is discussed further in Chapter 9) that is relevant to their practice in order to maintain and demonstrate current competence. The term competence according to the NMC (2010a) refers to the all-embracing set of knowledge, skills and attitudes essential to practise in a safe and effective manner without direct supervision. The NMC stipulates the competencies that are required for entry to the NMC register; these are generic competencies as well as field-specific competencies.

Queensland Nursing Council (2009) has its own definition of competence as 'the combination of skills, knowledge and attitudes, values and technical abilities that underpin safe and effective nursing practice and interventions'.

In the UK the competencies are acquired in stages that occur throughout the pre-registration nursing programme. It is a requirement that there is evidence that demonstrates that all competencies have been acquired and this evidence is used to establish whether a student is competent to practise as a nurse.

It must be remembered that each registered nurse and midwife is accountable for his or her actions and omissions (NMC, 2015). Accountability can never be delegated to any other person.

Lack of competence

Lack of competence is related to a lack of knowledge, skill or judgement of such a type that the nurse is unfit to practise in a safe way. Those nurses who have been deemed competent and fit to practise should posses the requisite skills, experience and qualifications relevant to the part of the professional register they have joined; they should be able to demonstrate a commitment to keeping those skills up to date and provide a service that is competent, safe, knowledgeable,

Table 3.3 Examples of lack of competence.

- There is a lack of skill or knowledge
- There is evidence of poor judgement
- The nurse is unable to work as part of a team
- The nurse has difficulty in communicating with colleagues or people in his or her care

understanding and focused completely on the needs of people in their care. Some examples of lack of competence are outlined in table 3.3.

If the nurse makes or continues to make errors or demonstrates poor practice over a prolonged period of time this can be deemed lack of competence. Despite the fact that a training need was identified and a supervised support programme was offered for the nurse, if their work only showed a temporary improvement which was not sustained when the programme was completed this could be grounds for considering lack of competence.

Other issues to be taken into account when considering incompetence include the nurse's ability. It might also be that the nurse continually demonstrates a lack of ability in correctly or appropriately calculating, administering and recording the administration or disposal of medications according to local policy and the standards issued by the NMC (2010b). There may be a persistent lack of ability in identifying the needs of people and as such there is inappropriate planning or delivery of care. The nurse may show lack of insight into their lack of competence. It should be remembered that attitude and character are just as important as competence. It is feasible to deliver care that is clinically skilled but if uncaring in this case, the nurse can also be deemed to lack competence.

Induction

Trust induction provides the new member of staff with information that is needed to help staff settle into their new place of work more quickly and safely. Induction is usually a mandatory requirement and forms a part of the person's contract of employment. Staff are required to attend the Trust induction which usually lasts for a day and consists of a series of presentations that are face to face as well as web-based e-learning activities for staff to complete. Regardless of the fact that you may well have been undertaking clinical placements at the trust where you are now working, your role now is different and you will be required to undertake induction. Table 3.4 outlines some of the lectures and sessions that are usually covered during trust induction.

Table 3.4 Induction day – core components.

- Welcome to the organisation
- Partnership working
- Personal safety (security)
- Clinical and organisational governance (quality)
- Self-care (looking after the whole person)
- Legal issues
- Security first (including data protection)
- Infection prevention and control (including hand washing)
- Customer care

Table 3.5 e-Learning packages that may be available as part of trust induction programmes.

- IT skills (some organisations use the European Computer Driving License)
- Fire safety
- Manual handling
- Use of equipment
- Working with hazardous substances
- Prevention of falls
- Infection prevention and control
- Use of personal protective equipment
- Various levels of life support (resuscitation)
- Managing data
- Data protection
- Vulnerability

e-Learning

e-Learning has become more popular in recent years for a number of reasons and much of the induction programme is now completed online using a variety of web-based e-learning materials. Those attending the induction day are required to undertake some preparation prior to commencing the e-learning; this is often needed as evidence of completion of the various packages (see table 3.5).

Auditing of the completion of the e-learning element of the trust induction programme is undertaken usually on a random basis, as those who successfully complete are provided with completion certificates for each module. These will be used for discussion with line managers, placed on the person's personnel file, updated on the individual training record and used at appraisal. There may be some constraints placed on the order in which the e-learning modules are undertaken and this should be ascertained prior to commencement.

Skills passport

Skills passports are often used in the pre-registration nursing programme. They are used to provide evidence to inform the assessment of Essential Skills Clusters and Standards of Proficiency while in the learning environment (NMC, 2010a) on an ongoing basis throughout the programme of study.

As a newly qualified nurse the organisation where you are employed may also make use of a skills passport. The skills being assessed will be different from those in the pre-registration programme but the way they are assessed (to deem competence) are similar. The skills are those that are identified as being central to the role of a nurse and are context dependent.

The skills passport is usually used in the first year after the nurse has qualified and is to be used alongside each person's preceptorship programme. It should be a structured process helping to ensure that key landmarks in the first year are being met. It provides an opportunity to enable the nurse to determine how he or she is developing and what is expected of him or her in the first post-qualifying year.

The organisation where you work may require you to demonstrate competence in a particular or a range of skills within a number of weeks of commencing employment, which may encompass mandatory and statutory training. Table 3.6 provides information concerning a range of activities that some trusts may require newly qualified nurses to undertake and be deemed competent in.

Things to consider

Using your preceptor as a 'learning tool' – they can often give you advice or information with experiences you may face; they have stood in your shoes.

Tapping into a more senior colleague's knowledge – using their wisdom can only help you develop your own professional know-how, competence and confidence.

Conclusion

From the moment they are registered, nurses are autonomous and accountable for their actions and omissions. Preceptorship is an activity that is associated with the provision of support and guidance offered during the early months of the nurse's career or when the nurse's role changes substantially. The process of

Table 3.6 Examples of a number of activities that some trusts may require newly qualified nurses to undertake and be deemed competent in with time limits.

Date	Activity
In the first 2 weeks of commencing employment	Mandatory training (including trust induction) This may be profession specific or generic
Within the first 6 months of commencing a new post	• Fundamentals of electrocardiography • Peripheral intravenous administration • Vital life support Updates every 2 years Intravenous administration updates as directed
To be completed at 6–9 months in post	• Central line catheter insertion • Catheterisation • Acute Life Events Recognition and Treatment (ALERT) • Awareness Why Anticipating and Responding is Essential (AWARE)
When 12 months in post	• Mentorship • Other courses appropriate to level of expertise and area of care

preceptorship is focused around enhancing and maximising the nurse's skills for the benefit of the patient, the individual and the organisation.

The period after registration with the NMC on completion of an education programme can be a challenging time; good support and guidance during this period is vital. Newly registered nurses who manage the transition successfully are able to provide effective care more quickly, feel more confident about their role and are more likely to remain within the profession. This means they are able to make a greater contribution to care, as well as ensuring that the benefits from the investment in their education is fully utilised.

References

DeCicco, J. (2008) "Developing a Preceptorship/Mentorship Model for Home Health Care Nurses". Journal of Community Health Nursing, Vol 25, No 1, pp. 15–25.

Department of Health (2010) "Preceptorship Framework for Newly Registered Nurses, Midwives and Allied Health Professionals". DH: London.

Nursing and Midwifery Council (2006) "Preceptorship Guidelines" NMC Circular 21/2006 SAT/gl October 3 2006.

Nursing and Midwifery Council (2010a) "Standards for Pre registration Nursing Education" http://standards.nmc-uk.org/PreRegNursing/statutory/background/Pages/introduction.aspx last (accessed June 2014).

Nursing and Midwifery Council (2010b) "Standards for Medicines Management" http://www.nmc-uk.org/Documents/NMC-Publications/NMC-Standards-for-medicines-management.pdf last (accessed June 2014).

Nursing and Midwifery Council (2015) "The Code. Professional Standards of Practice and Behaviour for Nurses and Midwives" http://www.nmc-uk.org/Documents/NMC-Publications/NMC-Code-A5-FINAL.pdf last (accessed January 2015).

Queensland Nursing Council (2009) "Scope of Practice – Framework for Nurses and Midwives" http://www.health.qld.gov.au/parrot/html/documents/nursingscprac.pdf last (accessed June 2014).

Robinson, S. and Griffiths, P. (2009) "Scoping Review. Preceptorship for Newly Qualified Nurses: Impacts, Facilitators and Constraints" http://www.kcl.ac.uk/nursing/research/nnru/publications/Reports/PreceptorshipReview.pdf last (accessed June 2014).

CHAPTER 4

Accountability and delegation

Aim

The aim of this chapter is to highlight the importance that accountability plays in providing care that is safe, effective and appropriate.

Objectives

By the end of this chapter you will be able to:
1. Explain the terms accountability and responsibility
2. Discuss accountability and decision making in relation to safe and effective practice
3. Demonstrate an understanding of appropriate delegation
4. Describe the principles underpinning delegation

Introduction

Accountability is and should be a key concern for nurses. Professional accountability entails being responsible for actions and for the outcomes of those actions. Accountability forms part of the framework of clinical governance, which provides safe, good quality, cost-effective, evidence-based care. Accountability is sometimes associated with blame and while being called to account for actions (and omissions) it may seem as if the nurse is being blamed; accountability should be more about empowering the nurse and ultimately the patient.

Accountability and responsibility

Nursing is a dynamic, complex and developing profession and this brings with it an increase in autonomy as well as an increase in accountability. As accountable

---

The Essential Guide to Becoming a Staff Nurse, First Edition. Ian Peate.
© 2016 John Wiley & Sons, Ltd. Published 2016 by John Wiley & Sons, Ltd.

practitioners, nurses must be able to clarify and explain why they have made the decisions they have as part of their practice. It is unacceptable to say 'I was just following orders'; ignorance of the law is no defence. Understanding what accountability is and is not along with its implications for practice will go some way to ensure that nurses will continue to expand and develop their practice when responding to patient and professional needs in a safe, competent and effective manner.

Accountability is not responsibility, but the two are very closely inter-twined – they go hand in hand. Nurses take responsibility for the care that they provide and they are also required to answer for their own decisions and actions. The nurse carries out these actions having agreed them with the patient, and if appropriate with the patient's families, their carers; they do this in such a way that they meet the obligations made of them by the NMC and the law.

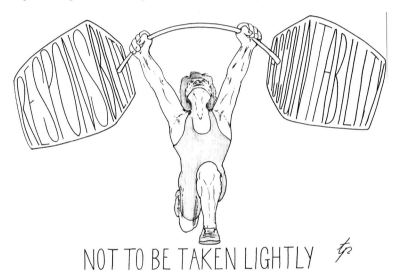

NOT TO BE TAKEN LIGHTLY

Working boundaries between health care practitioners are changing and registered nurses are taking on a number of tasks that had previously been undertaken by those working in the medical field, as well as this health care support workers are assuming responsibility for tasks and activities that had hitherto only been performed by registered nurses. As a result of this, issues concerning governance, risk management and legal accountability have and will continue to rise (Cox, 2011).

Rapid change is occurring in health and social care organisations in the UK with regard to restructuring and the delivery of services in order to offer the most efficient and effective care to service users. There have been a number of

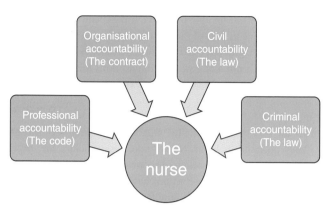

Figure 4.1 Spheres of accountability.

drivers that have led to a rethink with regard to roles and responsibilities for registered nurses as well as support workers with respect to the number and the scope of activities being carried out. This leads to consideration of the important issue of delegation and the associated issues of accountability and supervision.

Nurses and health service providers are accountable to both the criminal and civil courts to ensure that their activities are in alignment with legal requirements in the country that they are practising, as is the case with any other public body. As well as this, it is also important to note that employees are accountable to their employer and as such must abide by and follow their contract of employment. Nurses and other registered practitioners are also accountable to regulatory and professional bodies with regard to terms of standards of practice and patient care (The Code of Conduct NMC, 2015). Currently, not all support workers are subject to professional registration. Figure 4.1 provides an overview of the spheres of accountability.

Things to consider

In order to fully understand accountability:
- At all times make the patient your first concern
- Know the NMC Code
- Seek support when unsure and communicate
- Be responsive to comments made about you, criticisms and compliments
- Be a critical thinker
- Police yourself.

The code

Nurses are accountable professionally to their regulatory body, the NMC, which is in turn overseen by the Professional Standards Authority. The prime responsibility of the NMC is the protection of the public. It ensures that the nurse acts in an appropriate manner by reference to *The Code of Conduct* (NMC, 2015). The Code is not law, but is used by the NMC to establish if the nurse has performed in a manner that meets professional expectations.

The contract

From a contractual perspective the nurse is accountable to the employer. Within contracts of employment there is an implied term that employees will obey the reasonable instructions of their employers and that they will exercise all reasonable skill and care. Furthermore, most contracts will contain clauses that make it a condition of employment that the employee will abide by the policies and procedures that the employers have or will implement. If an employee fails to act within the terms of a contract of employment this may lead to termination or other sanctions.

The law

Nurses are accountable to society through the law and society can show its disapproval for certain acts through the use of criminal law. There are occasions where this sanction has been applied to nurses whose standards of care and performance have been so poor that this has led to serious harm taking place.

Over to you staff nurse

Have a look at your contract of employment and in this determine if there is any evidence to demonstrate that you are accountable to your employer. Look for implicit and explicit terms.

Delegation, accountability and responsibility

As you step into your new role there are going to be many challenging situations; one of the most challenging aspects of your new role may be how best to delegate tasks to support workers. This is an area of the role that many newly qualified nurses often struggle with.

Often it is usually you, the registered nurse, who is in overall charge of the nursing care of the patient. However, the nurse cannot undertake every aspect of care or task for every patient and as such there will be a need to delegate elements of that care to others.

NHS Wales (2010) define delegation as the process by which you (the delegator) allocate clinical or non-clinical treatment or care to a competent person (the delegatee). You will remain responsible for the overall management of the service user and accountable for your decision to delegate. You will not be accountable for the decisions and actions of the delegatee.

Over to you staff nurse

Nurses sometimes find it difficult to delegate. Consider how effective you are at delegating the work that can be delegated.

- Are there any tasks that you could delegate in order to provide more effective patient care?
- List the tasks that you could delegate.
- Who do you delegate tasks to and why?
- When you have delegated tasks who is accountable for the delegated activities?
- Do you feel comfortable when you are delegating?

Delegation is the process by which a registered nurse allocates work to a support worker who is considered competent to carry out the delegated task. The support worker then takes the responsibility for carrying out the delegated task. It should be noted that there is a difference between delegation and assignment. In delegation the support worker is responsible while the registered nurse retains accountability. In the assignment both the responsibility and accountability for an activity passes from one person to the other (Royal College of Speech and Language Therapists et al., RCSLT, 2006).

Selecting tasks or roles that are to be undertaken by support staff is a complex professional activity and should never be undertaken lightly and is dependent on the registered nurse's professional opinion; for any particular task, there are no general rules. It is essential to take into account the competence of the support worker with regard to the activity to be delegated.

Support workers in many settings across the United Kingdom are undertaking a number of disparate duties; they can be working at a range of levels that have come about as a result of delegation. The decision as to which activities are suitable to delegate sits squarely with the registered nurse who is always responsible for delegating the work to the support worker. It should be noted that there is no specific guidance regarding the activities that can or cannot be delegated.

Generally, the law does not prescribe who might perform particular health care tasks or roles; however, there are exceptions. Cox (2011) provides an example and notes that under mental health legislation, only doctors are authorised to carry out certain compulsory mental health care procedures. However, the law does insist that there is a standard of care related to each task or role that applies, regardless of who carries out the task. If the nurses extend or develop their role,

---

Over to you staff nurse

Think about a time when somebody had delegated a task or an activity to you. Consider the following:

- The person you were caring for and if they had confidence in you.
- The activity that was delegated to you.
- Your abilities and your confidence.
- How did you know how well you had performed in carrying out the activity?
- Having carried out that activity did you think there were areas that you needed to develop further?
- Did you feel supported?
- Did you take time to reflect on how well you performed?

---

they must be confident however that when they accept responsibility for the care of a patient they possess the knowledge, skills and experience that are required to perform the task or role to the requisite legal standard.

Things to consider

For you to delegate effectively and with confidence, it is essential that you understand the skill set of other members of the multidisciplinary team. Get to know the people you work with.

When delegating work to others, the nurse has a legal responsibility to have assessed the knowledge and skill level required to undertake the task being delegated (Mackey and Nancarrow, 2005). While the nurse is accountable for delegating the task to the delegatee (e.g. the support worker), the support worker is also accountable for accepting and taking on the delegated task; he or she is also responsible for the actions taken in carrying it out. This is the case if the support worker possesses the skills, knowledge and judgement to undertake the delegation and that the delegation of task falls within any guidelines and protocols within the workplace, as well as ensuring that the level of supervision and feedback is appropriate (see table 4.1).

Things to consider

Delegation is not about abdicating your duties; it is about working with and through other people.

Table 4.1 Some terms commonly used in the area of delegation.

Acceptable	Able to be agreed on; suitable
Accountability	The state of being answerable to a particular party, by rules or an organisational structure, for one's decisions and actions
Appropriate	Suitable or proper in the circumstances
Assignment	A task or piece of work allocated to someone as part of a job
Capability	The power or ability to do something
Capacity	The ability or power to do or understand something
Competence	The knowledge, skills, attitudes and ability to practise safely and effectively without the need for direct supervision
Competencies	Specific knowledge, skills, judgement and personal attributes needed for a health care professional to practice safely and ethically in a designated role and setting
Competent	Having the necessary ability, knowledge or skill to undertake something successfully
Consent	Permission for something to happen or agreement to do something
Delegate	Entrust a task or responsibility to another person, often one who is less senior than oneself
Delegatee	The person being delegated to
Delegation	The assignment of authority and responsibility to another person to carry out specific activities. Ultimate responsibility cannot be delegated – the delegator retains accountability for the delegation
Delegator	The person performing the delegation
Dependable	Trustworthy and reliable
Obligation	An act or course of action to which a person is morally, legally, religiously or institutionally bound; a duty or commitment
Performance	Competence in action
Policy	A plan or course of action, particularly one of an organisation or government
Protocol	The accepted or established code of procedure or behaviour in any group, organisation or situation
Referral	An act of referring someone or something for consultation, review or further action
Reliable	Consistently good in quality or performance; able to be trusted
Responsible	Having an obligation to do something, or having control over or care for someone, as part of your job or role. Morally accountable for one's behaviour
Scope of practice	The sphere of a person's profession in which he or she has the knowledge, skills and experience to practise safely and effectively in such a manner that meets the standards of their respective regulator and/or their employer and does not bring with it any risk to the public or to the health professional
Supervision	The active process of directing, guiding and influencing the outcome of a person's performance of a task
Task	An aspect of work to be carried out or undertaken

Source: Adapted from NHS Wales (2010) and The Chartered Society of Physiotherapy (2005).

Principles of delegation

The NMC has issued information to help nurses and midwives understand the matters surrounding delegation (NMC, 2012); the information should be read in conjunction with The Code (NMC, 2015). The information sets out principles for nurses to follow when they delegate duties to non-regulated health care staff with the aim of clarifying best practice. The principles focus on the interests of the patient, the role of the employers in the delegation process and when it is appropriate to refuse to allocate tasks to other health workers. The ability to delegate, assign tasks and supervise is a key skill for all registered nurses in any sphere of practice. All decisions associated with delegation by registered nurses have to be based on the fundamental tenets of safety and public protection. When nurses are thinking about which tasks and activities they are to delegate they should consider the principles outlined in table 4.2.

Things to consider

If others are delegating tasks to you (and they will), remember you also have a duty to determine if you have the appropriate knowledge and skills to accept this delegated activity. If you are unhappy about carrying out this activity, maybe because you do not have the knowledge and training in this area, you should always have the health and well-being of the patient at the forefront of your mind. Remember:

• Understand what it is you are specifically being asked to do.
• Determine if you have the appropriate training, knowledge and skills to undertake the task safely.
• Know how to get support should you need it.

Assessing needs and delegating

When assessing the needs of patients the initial assessment is usually a diagnostic one that relies on clinical reasoning and this requires the registered nurse (the assessor) to then formulate a plan of care. The registered nurse is expected to make the clinical (nursing) diagnosis, analyse and interpret the data amassed from assessment, and in partnership with the patient, formulate a plan of care and establish therapeutic options.

While working towards the aims (goals or objectives) that have been set by the registered practitioner the support worker will, however, be expected to make decisions within the context of the designated work with a patient. This applies to whether the support worker is performing tasks such as washing a patient or undertaking more complex activities. Regardless of the task, in both cases there is

Table 4.2 The principles associated with delegation.

- The key reason for delegation is to serve the interests of the patient/client
- The registered nurse carries out appropriate assessment, planning, implementation and evaluation of the delegated role
- The person to whom the task is delegated must have the appropriate role, level of experience and competence to carry it out
- Registered nurses must not delegate tasks and responsibilities to others that are beyond their level of skill and experience
- The support worker should undertake training to ensure competency in completing any tasks required. Training should be provided by the employer
- The task to be delegated is discussed and if the nurse and the support worker feel confident, the support worker can then carry out the delegated work/task
- The level of supervision and feedback provided is appropriate to the task being delegated. This should be based on the recorded knowledge and competence of the support worker, the needs of the patient, the service setting and the tasks assigned
- Regular supervision time is agreed and adhered to
- In multiprofessional settings, supervision arrangements may vary and will depend on the number of disciplines in the team and the line management structures of the registered practitioners
- The organisational structure has clearly defined lines of accountability and support workers are clear about their own accountability
- The support worker shares responsibility for raising any issues in supervision and can initiate discussion or request additional information and/or support
- The support worker will be required to make decisions within the context of a set of goals/care plan that have been negotiated with the patient and the health care team
- The support worker must at all times be aware of the extent of his or her expertise seeking support from available sources, when appropriate
- Documentation is completed by the appropriate person in accordance with employer's protocols and professional standards

Source: Adapted from NMC (2012), NHS Wales (2010) and Royal College of Speech and Language Therapists et al. (2006).

an opportunity for harm to occur. A duty of care applies and all staff have a duty of care and as such there is therefore a legal liability with respect to the person being cared for. Care that is provided must be competent and the person giving the care must perform in a competent manner. It is also important to remember that they have to inform another if they are unable to act competently.

The assessment phase is a part of the cyclical nursing process; it is a continuing aspect of the overall care plan. Therefore, support workers may be able to make judgements concerning patient progress and make some care decisions based on that judgement; they may assess and re-assess the patient's progress. The essential issue is that it is expected that a support worker who is delegated a task will be competent to continually monitor and evaluate changes in the patient responses to care interventions and to feedback appropriate information to the registered nurse.

Things to consider

Delegation is:
* Complex
* A concept
* An art that can be perfected as your experience grows
* A talent that requires effective impersonal skills
* A process that has to be followed through.

Where protocols have been formulated for an individual client group in a specific environment, it could be that the support worker may have delegated discretion, with limited and defined autonomy for some aspects of continual assessment. It is essential that the role and specific activities of the support worker are made clear in the formulation of such protocols. It is also essential that protocols are reviewed and up to date using the best available evidence.

Who should carry out the delegated activity?

Deciding who should carry out which delegated activity will depend on a variety of factors; there are three principal elements to be given consideration:

1 The individual's skills, competence, attitudes and experience of the health care provider(s)
2 The requirements of the patient group
3 The type of task in the specific context (hospital, community)

The delegation of activity is established in the context of the relationship that exists between the nurse delegating and the delegatee (see figure 4.2).

Several factors are important and should be thought about prior to deciding on whether to delegate a duty to a support worker. The nurse should consider that a support worker with a long service might be assumed to have developed substantial understanding of practice as a result of his or her day-to-day experience. Long service does not necessarily lead to the development of competence, just as undertaking a programme of education is not indicative of competence. However, some people can become extremely competent after working for only a short time in a particular sphere of practice. It is important, therefore, to assess the competence of individuals within the specific setting. It follows therefore

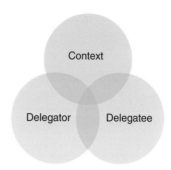

Figure 4.2 The delegating triumvirate.

that registered nurses must have the requisite skills to effectively carry out these assessments.

When assessing competence, the registered nurse should have an awareness and knowledge of the education, training and qualifications undertaken as well as knowing whether the support worker has previously performed a particular task competently. Training prior to delegation taking place may be needed if the support worker has not carried out the task before.

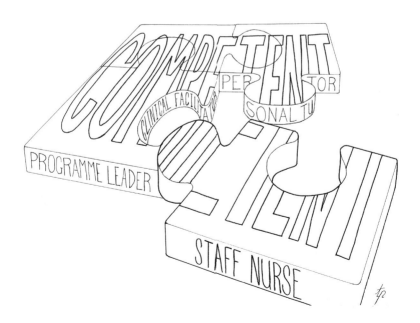

Recognised national qualifications allow individuals to demonstrate their competence by applying knowledge, understanding and skills to perform to the standards required in employment. The support worker would have had to have undertaken a formal assessment of practical competence with a knowledge base that underpins the practical aspects of their work.

Over to you staff nurse

Before delegating a task to a support worker, the following three questions need to be answered:

1 Do you think the support worker is competent to carry out the task(s)?
2 Does the support worker consider himself or herself to be competent to undertake the activity?
3 Does the task require an ongoing assessment of the patient to be made?

Source: Royal College of Nursing (2011).

Box 4.1 The principles of delegation.

- Delegation must always be in the best interest of the patient and not performed simply in an effort to save time or money.
- The support worker must have been suitably trained to perform the task.
- The support worker should always keep full records of training given, including dates.
- There should be written evidence of competence assessment, preferably against recognised standards such as National Occupational Standards; there should be clear guidelines and protocols in place so that the support worker is not required to make a clinical judgement that he or she is not competent to make.
- The role should be within the support worker's job description.
- The team and any support staff need to be informed that the task has been delegated (e.g. a receptionist in a GP surgery or ward clerk in a hospital setting).
- The person who delegates the task must ensure that an appropriate level of supervision is available and that the support worker has the opportunity for mentorship. The level of supervision and feedback provided must be appropriate to the task being delegated. This will be based on the recorded knowledge and competence of the support worker, the needs of the patient/client, the service setting and the tasks assigned.
- Ongoing development to ensure that competency is maintained is essential.
- The whole process must be assessed for the degree of risk.

Source: Royal College of Nursing (2011).

Supervising others

The registered nurse is responsible for formulating a system of supervision that aims to protect the patient as well as upholding the highest possible standards of care. This is closely aligned to the concept of clinical governance, accountability and responsibility. Clinical governance is defined by Scally and Donaldson (1998) as 'A framework through which NHS organisations are accountable for continuously improving the quality of their services and safe-guarding high standards of care by creating an environment in which excellence in clinical care will flourish'. There are said to be seven pillars of clinical governance:
1 Clinical effectiveness
2 Risk management
3 Patient experience and involvement
4 Communication
5 Resource effectiveness
6 Strategic effectiveness
7 Learning effectiveness.

Over to you staff nurse

How do you ensure that the person you are delegating an activity or task to:
- Understands what it is you are specifically asking them to do?
- Has the right training, knowledge and skills to take on that task safely and effectively?
- Knows how and where to get support if he or she needs it?

At the heart of clinical governance is patient safety and the management of risks; clinical governance is a part of everything nurses do and this includes the supervision of delegates (see figure 4.3). Ongoing supervision is required in order to assess the support worker's ability to carry out the delegated task and his or her capability to take on additional roles and responsibilities. It is advocated that a named supervisor is provided. The Royal College of Speech and Language Therapists et al. (2006) suggest that the following should apply:
- A system should be in place for support workers to access supervision and clinical advice as needed.
- Frequent supervision time is agreed between the registered practitioner and the support worker; a record is made of each session.
- The registered practitioner must have the required skills to support and assess the delegate (the supervisee).

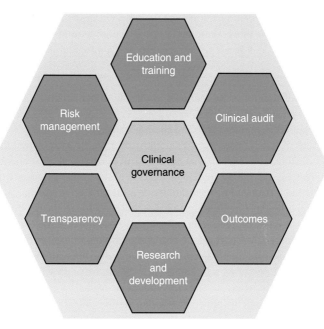

Figure 4.3 Clinical governance.

- The support worker shares responsibility for raising issues in supervision and may initiate discussion or request additional information/support.
- When the registered practitioner is absent from a setting where the support worker is working there should be an identified contact in case of query or emergency.

Supervision can vary in terms of what it includes. It can feature elements of direction, guidance, observation, joint working, discussion, exchange of ideas and coordination of activities. It may be direct or indirect, according to the type of the work being delegated. The decision regarding the amount and type of supervision needed is based on the registered practitioner's professional judgement and is determined by the recorded knowledge and competence of the support worker, the needs of the patient, the service setting and the task being delegated. The following factors should be considered by the registered practitioner and include:

- The level of experience and understanding of the support worker appropriate to the task being delegated
- Assessment of the support worker's competence relevant to the delegated task
- The complexity of the delegated tasks
- The stability and predictability of the patient's condition

- The care environment or setting and the support infrastructure available (e.g. whether working in a community, acute or school setting)
- Availability of and access to support from an appropriate registered professional(s)
- Periodic review of the patient's outcomes
- An identified process for periodic review and evaluation of the support worker's performance
- A recognised system for recording and reporting.

Appraisal of the support worker's performance, particularly where this process is linked to assessing personal development needs, offers a useful means by which the manager and the individual member of staff can ascertain any training needs, define learning outcomes and decide on what kind of learning activity is the most appropriate. Supervision and appraisal can support the development of individuals in line with personal need and service requirements.

Support workers, under the supervision of registered nurses, are now delivering a considerable amount of hands-on care. It must be remembered that support workers are not registered staff and as such they must be provided with appropriate training and where possible this should be aligned to national standards. Patients have the right to know who is caring for them and they should be able to anticipate that those who are providing their care are knowledgeable and competent. Support workers need to feel confident of their abilities in changing environments and registered nurses need to feel confident in delegating activities to support workers (Royal College of Speech and Language Therapists et al., 2006).

Things to consider

Delegation requires
- Confidence
- Management skills
- Mentorship skills
- Knowledge and understanding of the multidisciplinary team
- Awareness of scope of practice
- Knowledge and understanding of professional and legal liabilities.

Conclusion

Developing further understanding of accountability and related issues is vital as you begin your career; these issues are central to all that the nurse does. Exploring the issues discussed in this chapter may help you to address gaps in continuing professional development and promote the purpose of accountability.

Nurses are accountable for the decision to delegate care. The delegatee should know his or her limitations and know when to seek advice from the appropriate professional in the event that events change. If these conditions have been met and an aspect of care is delegated, the delegatee becomes accountable for his or her actions and decisions. Where another person, for example, an employer, has the authority to delegate an aspect of care, then it is the employer who becomes accountable for that delegation.

The people you offer care to should expect the same standard of care, regardless of who delivers it. When you delegate any aspect of care, you have a duty to determine that delegation is always in the best interest of the patient. You should remember that the person delegating the task is accountable for the appropriateness of the delegation. If you have made the decision that the delegation of a task to another person is appropriate, then the support worker is accountable for the standard of performance. The level of supervision offered has to be appropriate to the situation and must take into account the complexity of the task, the competence of the support worker and the needs of the patient as well as the setting in which the care is being delivered.

References

Cox, C. (2011) "Legal Responsibility and Accountability". Nursing Management, Vol 17, No **3**, pp. 18–20.

Mackey, H. and Nancarrow, S. (2005) "Assistant Practitioners: Issues of Accountability, Delegation and Competence". International Journal of Therapeutic Rehabilitation, Vol 12, No **8**, pp. 331–338.

NHS Wales (2010) "All Wales Guideline for Delegations" http://www.wales.nhs.uk/ sitesplus/861/opendoc/181978 last (accessed June 2013).

Nursing and Midwifery Council (2012) "Delegation" http://www.nmc-uk.org/Nurses-and-midwives/advice-by-topic/a/advice/Delegation/ last (accessed June 2013).

Nursing and Midwifery Council (2015) "The Code. Professional Standards of Practice and Behaviour for Nurses and Midwives" http://www.nmc-uk.org/Documents/NMC-Publications/NMC-Code-A5-FINAL.pdf last (accessed January 2015).

Royal College of Nursing (2011) "Accountability and Delegation: What You Need to Know" http://www.rcn.org.uk/__data/assets/pdf_file/0003/381720/003942.pdf last (accessed June 2013).

Royal College of Speech and Language Therapists et al (2006) "Supervision, Accountability and Delegation of Activities to Support Workers". RCSLT: London.

Scally, G. and Donaldson, L.J. (1998) "Looking Forward: Clinical Governance and the Drive for Quality Improvement in the New NHS in England". British Medical Journal, Vol 317, pp. 61–65.

The Chartered Society of Physiotherapy (2005) "Physiotherapy Competence and Capability Resource Pack". CSP: London.

CHAPTER 5

Using the evidence

Aim

The aim of this chapter is to develop further an understanding of how to apply research skills and knowledge in the workplace.

Objectives

By the end of this chapter you will be able to:
1 Define evidence-based practice (EBP)
2 Distinguish between EBP and research
3 Understand how the use of an evidence base can enhance care provision and safety
4 Explain how evidence can be incorporated into nursing practice
5 Discuss the challenges associated with the implementation of EBP

Introduction

There have been and will continue to be a number of changes in health care and the ways in which it is provided. The nurse has to be comfortable in adopting to change as well as being able to welcome change and challenges in order to ensure that care provision is safe and based on sound evidence.

Spending on health and social care has been on the rise for many years and one aspect of the role of the nurse is to reduce health care costs, at the same time ensuring that care provision is not compromised. Specific efforts are being made by government and individual organisations to reduce costs; these include the ways in which care is managed, ensuring staffing levels are appropriate (not just numbers but skill mix also), improving the retention of staff, the use of information technology (including the electronic health care

The Essential Guide to Becoming a Staff Nurse, First Edition. Ian Peate.
© 2016 John Wiley & Sons, Ltd. Published 2016 by John Wiley & Sons, Ltd.

record), reducing the number of patient care errors and the effective use of evidence-based care.

Over to you staff nurse

Take some time to think about an everyday element of your practice, such as thromboembolic prophylaxis, percutaneous endoscopic gastrostomy (PEG) feeding or the use of oxygen. What is it that informs your practice? What are your actions and those of your colleagues mostly based on – are they based on research findings, clinical guidelines or intuition?

In all of our lives, in our homes and in our places of work errors abound. Patients and clinicians are affected by near errors and the consequences of adverse events on an hourly basis. The effects of health care errors and poor quality health care have impacted all our lives, directly and indirectly.Patient safety and quality care are at the heart of health care systems and processes in place to achieve this are reliant on nurses. To achieve goals in patient safety and quality and as such enhance health care, nurses must assume the leadership role. The imperative to improve the quality and safety of care is the concern of all clinicians, all health care providers as well as all health care leaders and managers.

It is crucial that all nurses engage in lifelong learning, using data and information as well as research evidence to inform their practice. Along with experiential knowledge, analyses and evidence, the nurse is challenged to continuously improve care processes and to encourage others to ensure that those who are in receipt of our care receive the best possible care, irrespective of their ethnicity or gender, where it is that they live or their socioeconomic status.

There are various issues and factors that come together to define the complexity and scope of patient safety and the provision of quality care along with a need to provide various strategies to create change within health care systems and care provision. Providing care that uses the best available evidence can lead to an improvement in quality and safety, leading to better care for the people we offer care to.

Using research and implementing the evidence are activities you are very familiar with. Your undergraduate nursing programme would have exposed you to these important aspects of professional practice. As you progress in your chosen field you will continue to develop the skills associated with research and the importance of providing care that has an evidence base.

Things to consider

To be successful with EBP, nurses have to be willing to challenge their own assumptions and be willing to work with others with the intention of improving care provision and patient outcomes.

Definitions of terms

The term 'evidence-based medicine' began to emerge during the 1980s describing the approach that used scientific evidence to establish best practice. The term then became 'evidence-based practice' (EBP) as other clinicians apart from doctors acknowledged the importance of scientific evidence when making clinical decisions. A number of definitions of EBP have emerged in the literature, but the most commonly used definition comes from Sackett et al. (1996) who suggest that EBP concerns the integration of clinical expertise and the best available evidence from systematic research; they also note that it involves the careful and well thought through use of current best evidence concerning the care of individuals. When nurses and health care professionals use an evidence base this can help reduce ritual and isolated haphazard clinical experiences along with practice where there is no foundation, which is often based on an individual's opinion, hearsay, custom and practice.

Experts then began to talk about evidence-based health care as a process by which research evidence is applied in making decisions about an explicit population or a group of patients. EBP and evidence-based health care make the assumption that evidence is used in the context of a particular patient's preferences and desires, the clinical situation as well as the expertise of the clinician. It is also expected that health care professionals can read, critique and combine research findings and interpret existing evidence-based clinical practice guidelines.

Using an evidence base according to Walsh and Wigens (2003) provides an advantage for health care professionals as the knowledge base of individuals grows and improves and they are able to demonstrate an increase in confidence when making clinical decisions. Zerwekh and Garneau (2014) add that EBP is one strategy that can be used to reduce the amount of time needed to integrate new health care findings into practice.

Muir Gray (1997) has described EBP as 'doing the right things right'. It is a method of problem-solving used to produce the best solution and a combination of clinical expertise with application to the best available evidence from systematic research.

Evidence-based practice, research and quality improvement

EBP is not research utilisation, quality improvement or nursing research, yet it can be associated with each of these processes. Quality improvement projects may be evidence based, and the findings can influence other EBP or research initiatives. An EBP project can lead to a research study or a quality improvement initiative. Nurses have used the research available to guide nursing practice and to improve patient outcomes; this involves critical analysis and evaluation of research findings, determining how they fit into clinical practice. Research utilisation is being replaced by EBP.

Quality improvement focuses on systems, processes and functions, clinical, satisfaction and financial outcomes. Quality improvement efforts are not usually intended to develop nursing practice standards or to advance the science of nursing; however, they may add to an understanding of best practices. Quality improvement, in health care, is not meant to produce scientific knowledge; rather it serves as a management tool to advance the processes and outcomes within a particular setting.

Quality improvement initiatives are often concerned with addressing clinical problems or issues, examining processes and using specific markers to assist in the evaluation of clinical performance. Data are collected and then analysed to assist with understanding the process and the related outcomes; findings help contribute to efforts to attain and sustain continuous improvement through ongoing monitoring and improvement activities.

EBP is the use of research from professional experts that looks at the patient's preferences, uses clinical expertise and integrates the best evidence. Research is a systematic inquiry that answers questions and solves problems; quality improvement improves work processes to improve patient outcomes.

Clinical governance focuses on reducing risk and enhancing people's quality of care. It is central to health care, and patient safety is the chief priority for all staff. Other terms that are synonymous with clinical governance include:
- Quality assurance
- Clinical audit
- Quality enhancement
- Clinical effectiveness
- EBP.

The NHS aims to offer a range of services that are responsive to individual and local needs and in order to do this effectively, they must decentralise its provision and become devolved. A way of making this move towards devolution is to change the way health services are managed and run. Centralised services have the potential to fail to provide patient-centred care and forget to acknowledge that patients are individuals with local and individual needs. Care has to be delivered in such a way that it is meaningful to those who pay for it – service users and the public.

Clinical governance aims to continuously improve, strengthen and build upon current systems of quality assurance across a range of services. There are several activities associated with clinical governance, including:

- Clinical audit
- Risk management
- Significant event audit
- EBP
- Reviewing complaints
- The involvement of users and carers
- Professional development.

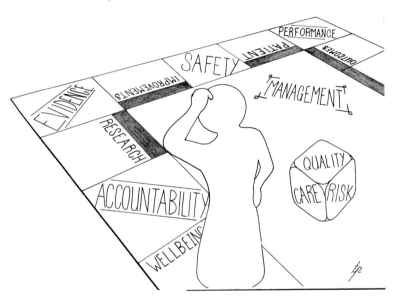

If clinical governance is to be effective, then there are a number of points that must be considered: primarily it must focus on the improvement of the quality of patient care and this has to be applied to all areas where care takes place. The nature of interprofessional working and the partnerships that exist not only among staff but also between staff and patients must be given consideration. Public and patient involvement is an important prerequisite for effective clinical governance; feedback from users of the services can promote a culture that recognises mistakes, acts upon them and provides feedback. This applies to all health care staff but nurses have a particular role to play as a result of their evidence-based professional practice and their central role in influencing the patient's experience. Using the many facets of clinical governance, nurses can focus on the needs of the people they offer care to, aiming to constantly evaluate and improve patient care.

Clinical governance cannot be achieved in isolation; structures need to be in place to support it, as well as ensuring that there are common standards and the common public ethos is ensured. There are national structures in place to support local clinical governance initiatives; in England, for example, this is the Care Quality Commission (CQC). The CQC aims to ensure that health and social care services provide people with safe, effective, compassionate, high-quality care as well as encouraging service improvements. Their role is to inspect and regulate services in order to apply performance ratings to enhance patient choice (CQC, 2013).

Five stages of evidence-based practice

There are five stages associated with EBP (see figure 5.1).

1 **The questions**
   This stage is about asking answerable clinical questions. The first step is to recognise that there is a need for new information. The information needed at this stage is likely to be vague and because of this it will have to be converted into an answerable question with the aim of facilitating an effective search for the answer. You will only yield precise answers when you have provided a precise question; a specific question has to be asked. The question should be carefully framed, as this helps determine what type of evidence you will need to locate. It could be that a number of questions will emerge at the same time – this is not unusual; however, it will not be possible to answer all of them at once. Failure to ask a focused and precise clinical question can be a major threat to EBP; so this first stage needs to be given much thought.

   The question helps to explore the subject and focus on the right informa-tion to provide answers to the question. Wild (2014) suggests that an initial starting point could be questioning one's own practice and to consider why and how a decision about the treatment or care provided is made. PICO is a framework that can be used for formulating questions developed by Sackett et al. (1997) in order to make the question more focused:

   P – Population or Patient – specify gender, age, disease type, morbidity, stipulate the setting, such as, inpatient or surgical care for information that relates to the clinical environment

   I – Intervention – define what it is you are interested in; this could be a test or exposure to something (e.g. chemicals)

   C – Comparison – define an alternative intervention by means of comparison

   O – Outcomes – define the meaningful outcome if this is beneficial or harmful.

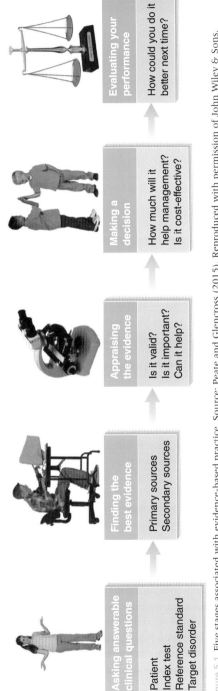

Asking answerable clinical questions	Finding the best evidence	Appraising the evidence	Making a decision	Evaluating your performance
Patient Index test Reference standard Target disorder	Primary sources Secondary sources	Is it valid? Is it important? Can it help?	How much will it help management? Is it cost-effective?	How could you do it better next time?

Figure 5.1 Five stages associated with evidence-based practice. Source: Peate and Glencross (2015). Reproduced with permission of John Wiley & Sons.

2 **Obtaining the evidence, locating the evidence**

Choosing the right evidence is of highest importance. There are many different sources of evidence, and it can be hard to know where to begin (see figure 5.2 sources of evidence).

The main sources of evidence often come from more experienced colleagues and textbooks; however, there are difficulties with these sources of information. How can you be sure that the information that your colleagues provide is reliable?

Over to you staff nurse

What do you understand by the term anecdotal evidence? Is it appropriate to use anecdotal evidence to support your clinical practice and the clinical decision you make?

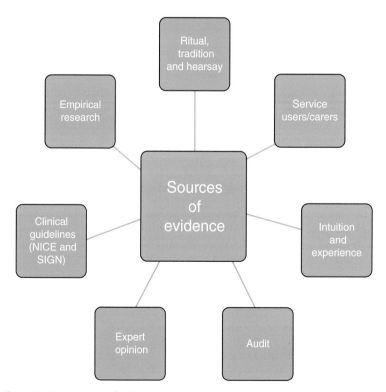

Figure 5.2 Some sources of evidence.

When you use the evidence from textbooks the opinions that are expressed could be out of date before the book has even been published, or it may be incompatible with current best available evidence. A number of groups have put together levels or hierarchies of evidence; these are usually based upon scientific merit in an empirical model. When examining the evidence it will be helpful if you consider the hierarchy of evidence identified in table 5.1.

The evidence can be found in:
○ Books
○ Journals
○ The Internet
○ Reports
○ Electronic data bases (e.g. internurse, CINAHL, Science Direct, OVID).

When retrieving evidence, a reliable source is to use a systematic review that summarises the results from a large amount of high-quality research studies. The first place to check for reviews in health care is The Cochrane Library.

Over to you staff nurse

Log on to the Cochrane Collection web site at www.cochrane.org. Locate the top 50 reviews, choose one of them and read it. Having read the review did you find the information in the list of value to your practice setting? If so why and if not why?

Table 5.1 Hierarchy of evidence.

Level	Description of evidence	Strength
I	Systematic review or meta-analysis of all relevant randomised controlled trials (RCTs), or evidence-based clinical practice guidelines based on systematic reviews of RCTs	Strongest
II	Evidence from at least one well-designed RCT	
III	Evidence from well-designed controlled trials without randomisation	
IV	Evidence from well-designed case–control and cohort studies	
V	Systematic reviews of descriptive and qualitative studies	
VI	A single descriptive or qualitative study	
VII	The opinion of authorities and/or reports of expert committees	Weakest

Source: Adapted from Melnyk and Fineout-Overholt (2005).

The Cochrane Library is not a standard bibliographic database; this source is a collection of a variety of separate databases and is available as a CD-ROM and can also be accessed via the Internet. Most universities and health care providers have access to the Internet version.

Over to you staff nurse

How would you undertake a search for information concerning the care of women with breast cancer? Make a list of the sources you would go to; remember the sources have to be reliable.

3 Assessing the evidence – appraising

It is important to critically appraise the evidence in order to determine its validity and its potential worth. The following are key questions to ask when appraising the evidence:

- Can the evidence be trusted?
- What does the evidence mean?
- Does this answer the question?
- Is it relevant to practice?

There are different appraisal and interpreting skills that can be utilised; these are contingent upon the kind of evidence being considered. Table 5.2 outlines one of the many ways of appraising the evidence.

Table 5.2 One way of appraising the evidence.

- The report structure – is it logical in its progression?
- The abstract – does it offer the reader an insight into the theme of the study how it was conducted and the key findings?
- The introduction – does this explain the how and the why elements of the study?
- The purpose of the research – is this established from the beginning, with a rationale that is specific in order to address the study question?
- The literature review – how up to date is the literature that is being used in order to support the study and is it broad enough to provide a wide review?
- Methodology – does the methodology provide a step-by-step approach to the processes involved in the study?
- The analysis of the data – is there a complete discussion of the data that has been provided?
- The discussion – is this presented in a critical way?
- The conclusions and limitations – have the implications for practice been identified?
- References and bibliography – do those that have been used reflect the literature review and are they applicable to the study?

Source: Adapted from Burns and Grove (2011) and Polit and Beck (2011).

> **Over to you staff nurse**
>
> Having appraised the literature (using the various options open to you), you are asked to advise a woman who has recently undergone bilateral mastectomy on how to prevent infection at the incision. How would provide this information and why?

4 **Arriving at a decision – acting on evidence**

This step requires the nurse to apply the evidence to the individual patient and Del Mar et al. (2008) consider this to be the most difficult step. When you have arrived at a decision that the evidence is of sound quality, at this point another decision will have to be made and this is whether the evidence should be incorporated into clinical practice, and whether it should be used to implement change. Consideration of both the advantages and the risks inherent in implementing the change as well as the benefits and the risks of excluding any alternatives should be undertaken. These decisions must be made in partnership with members of the multidisciplinary team, managers and those who use the services where this is appropriate. Resistance to change must be given serious consideration, as resisting change can be a challenge. When involving all key stakeholders (e.g. colleagues, patients, carers, budget holders and commissioners) this can assist in ensuring that the change is implemented as well as sustained.

5 **Evaluation and reflection – evaluation of performance**

Evaluation and reflection are central when establishing if the action(s) taken have accomplished the anticipated results. This is a fundamental feature of health care practice.

EBP should be seen as a continuous, cyclical process. Once each stage of the process has been worked through then it is probable that new questions will surface and these too will need to be answered. EBP should focus on using a questioning approach to the care that you deliver. This should never be seen as a 'one-off' activity – it is a constant process that can assist in providing safe and high-quality care to the people you offer care to. An evidence-based approach can also help you with regard to your own professional development in so far as you question and seek evidence-based solutions.

Integrating evidence-based practice into care delivery

It should not be assumed that effective clinical practice is based on the best possible, rigorously tested evidence; this is not always the case. EBP is difficult to avoid in contemporary nursing practice. The Code (NMC, 2015) requires the nurses to ensure that the care and any advice that they provide are based on the use of the best available evidence. All nurses and other health care professionals need to understand and contribute to the body of knowledge that is the foundation for their clinical practice. The nurse is accountable for determining the value of care interventions. EBP requires you to use current best evidence when you make decisions about care provision.

There are a number of organisations that also demand that practitioners use an evidence-based approach to the delivery of care apart from the NMC, for example, the CQC, whose job it is to check whether hospitals, care homes, GPs, dentists and other services are meeting national standards. This is an example of an external force that pushes health and social providers towards the development and maintenance of systems to find, appraise and disseminate best practices. Failure to comply with these requirements may mean that sanctions are applied to those organisations that are unable to demonstrate an evidence-based approach to care.

Challenges to implementation of evidence-based practice

There are several reasons why EBPs are the exception as opposed to the rule. EBP systems themselves may facilitate this while other barriers are concerned with human factors, and others related to the organisations within which patient care is provided. Table 5.3 identifies some common barriers to implementing evidence as a basis for practice.

Pagoto et al. (2007) have considered what health care professionals perceive to be both the barriers and facilitators of EBP. Seven themes have been identified to describe barriers and also the facilitators:

1 Training and educational support
2 Attitudes towards EBP and research
3 Consumer demand for evidence-based care
4 Logistical and organisational considerations
5 Institutional and leadership support
6 Policies and procedures
7 Access to appropriate evidence.

Failing to adopt an evidence-based approach to care can result in poor decision-making and this can then have a detrimental effect on a person's health and well-being. Applying EBP is associated with the management of change (Ellis, 2013). Change can take many years to occur from an idea to the implementation of that idea (NICE, 2007); understanding the barriers to change

Table 5.3 Factors that may impact on the implementation of EBP.

Barrier	Reasons
The EBP system itself	• Vast amount of information available in the literature
Human factors	• Lack of understanding concerning EBP • Insufficient skills required for finding and/or appraising the literature • Negativity about research and evidence-based care (for a number of reasons) • Apathy • Misperceptions that the use of evidence and research is only for medicine
Organisational factors	Lack of authority given to the nurse to make changes in practice Peer pressure 'we've always done it this way' Challenging workloads with little or no time for research activities Conflict in priorities Lack of administrative (or appropriate administrative) support Lack of organisational incentive

Source: Adapted from NICE (2007) and Houser (2011).

can help with this sometimes complex process. When the nurse does not use an evidence-based approach this has an adverse impact not only on the patient but also on the nurse. The Code (NMC, 2015) stipulates that the nurse must use up to date knowledge and evaluate care in order to assess, plan, deliver and evaluate care. Allegations of professional misconduct could be made if a nurse does not use an evidence base in practice.

Things to consider

Madsen et al. (2005) have published an evidence-based project that describes the potential benefits of stopping the accepted practice of listening to the bowel sounds of patients who have undergone elective abdominal surgery. The literature was reviewed and an assessment of current practice was undertaken; Madsen et al. (2005) reported that clinical parameters such as the return of flatus and first postoperative bowel movement were more helpful than bowel sounds in verifying the return of gastrointestinal mobility post abdominal surgery. This evidence-based project has resulted in saving nursing time without having any negative impact on patient outcomes.

Regardless of the barriers it is evident that nurses are embracing and engaging in EBP and are making a difference in patient outcomes. Fink et al. (2005) note that barriers can be overcome when organisational efforts are focused on integrating research in practice and using strategies such as journal clubs and nursing grand rounds and having research articles available for review.

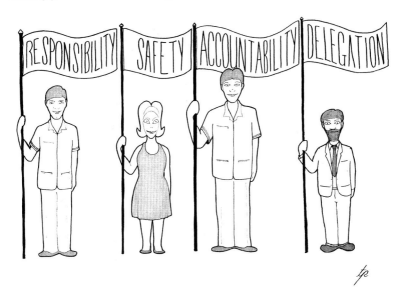

Conclusion

The science of translating research into practice is rather new; however, there is some guidance concerning what implementation interventions to use in enhancing patient safety when implementing care. It must be remembered however that there is no magic wand available that will change what is known from research into practice. To move evidence-based interventions into practice, a number of strategies are needed. Furthermore, what may work in one context of care may or may not work in another setting; as such, it is essential to remember that context variables count in implementation.

References

Burns, N. and Grove, S.K. (2011) (4th Ed) "Understanding Nursing Research". Elsevier: Philadelphia.

Care Quality Commission (2013) "Raising Standards, Putting People First. Our Strategy 2013–2016". Care Quality Commission: Newcastle upon Tyne.

Del Mar, C., Doust, J. and Glasziou, P. (2008) "Clinical Thinking. Evidence, Communication and Decision Making". Blackwell: Oxford.

Ellis, P. (2013) (2nd Ed) "Getting Evidence in to Practice", in Ellis, P. (Ed), "Evidence-Based Practice Nursing", Ch 8, pp. 124–142. Learning Matters: London.

Fink, R., Thompson, C. J. and Bonnes, D. (2005) "Overcoming Barriers and Promoting the Use of Research in Practice". Journal of Nursing Administration, Vol 35, No **3**, pp. 121–129.

Houser, J. (2011) "Evidence Based Practice in Healthcare", in Houser, J. and Oman, K.S. (Eds) "Evidence Based Practice. An Implementation Guide for Healthcare Organizations", Ch 1, pp. 1–19. Jones and Bartlett: Sudbury.

Madsen, D., Sebolt, T., Cullen, L., Folkedahl, B., Mueller, T., Richardson, C., et al. (2005). "Listening to Bowel Sounds: An Evidence-based Practice Project". American Journal of Nursing, Vol 105, No **12**, pp. 40–49.

Melnyk, B. and Fineout-Overholt, E. (2005) "Evidence Based Practice in Nursing and Healthcare: A Guide to Best Practice". Lippincott: Philadelphia.

Muir Gray, J.A. (1997) "Evidence-based Practice is About 'Doing the Right Things Right", in "Evidence-based Healthcare: How to Make Health Policy and Management Decisions". Churchill Livingstone: Edinburgh.

National Institute of Care and Health Excellence (2007) "How to Change Practice: Understand, Identify and Overcome Barriers to Change". NICE: London.

Nursing and Midwifery Council (2015) "The Code. Professional Standards of Practice and Behaviour for Nurses and Midwives" http://www.nmc-uk.org/Documents/NMC-Publications/NMC-Code-A5-FINAL.pdf last (accessed January 2015).

Pagoto, S., Spring, B., Coups, E., Mulvaney, S., Coutu, M. and Ozakinci, G. (2007) "Barriers and Facilitators of Evidence-based Practice Perceived by Behavioral Science Health Professionals". Journal of Clinical Psychology, Vol 63, No **7**, pp. 695–705.

Polit, D.F. and Beck, C.T. (2011) (9th Ed) "Nursing Research: Generating and Accessing Evidence in Nursing Practice". Lippincott: Philadelphia.

Sackett, D., Rosenburg, W., Gray, J. et al (1996) "Evidence Base Medicine: What it is and What it is Not". British Medical Journal, Vol 312, pp. 71–72.

Sackett, D.L., Richardson, W.S., Rosenburg, W. and Haynes, R.B. (1997) (2nd Ed) "Evidence-Based Medicine: How to Practise and Teach EBM". Churchill Livingstone: Edinburgh.

Walsh, M. and Wigens, L. (2003) "Introduction to Research". Nelson Thorne: Cheltenham.

Wild, K. (2014) "The Professional Nurse and Contemporary Health Care", in Peate, I., Wild, K. and Nair, M. (Eds) "Nursing Practice, Knowledge and Care", Ch 2, pp. 25–45. Wiley: Oxford.

Zerwekh, J. and Garneau, A. (2014) (7th Ed) "Nursing Today. Transitions and Trends". Elsevier: Philadelphia.

CHAPTER 6

Working with patients and their families

Aim

The aim of this chapter is to discuss the importance of working in partnership with patients and their families when providing health care.

Objectives

By the end of this chapter you will be able to:

1 Explain the advantages of working in partnership with patients and their families
2 Discuss the NHS Constitution
3 Outline the NHS complaints procedure
4 Distinguish between the various types of statements
5 Understand the component parts that make up a statement
6 Demonstrate insight into the many resources available

Introduction

When patients are engaged in their health care, it can lead to measurable improvements in safety and quality. The nurse is required to work in partnership with people as outlined in the Code of Conduct NMC (2015).

Patient engagement also incorporates shared decision making and is fundamentally about giving patients the opportunity to be active participants in their health care. When well-informed patients and caregivers work with health care professionals, it is more likely that patients will be recipients of care that meets their needs and see improved health outcomes; quality and safety will also improve.

The goal of patient and family engagement is to create an environment where patients, families, clinicians and other health care staff all work together as

---

The Essential Guide to Becoming a Staff Nurse, First Edition. Ian Peate.
© 2016 John Wiley & Sons, Ltd. Published 2016 by John Wiley & Sons, Ltd.

partners with the intention of improving the quality and safety of care provision. Working in partnership with patients brings the perspectives of patients and their families directly into the planning, delivery and evaluation of care.

Things to think about

The ultimate measure by which to judge the quality of a medical effort is whether it helps patients (and their families) as they see it. Anything done in health care that does not help a patient or family is, by definition, waste, whether or not the professions and their associations traditionally hallow it.

Berwick (1997)

Involving patients and families who receive health care offers insights and input to help those to whom we provide care and services that are based on patient and family-identified needs, as opposed to the assumptions of nurses, clinicians or other staff about what it is that patients and families want. We will be responding to the needs of those we have the privilege to care for.

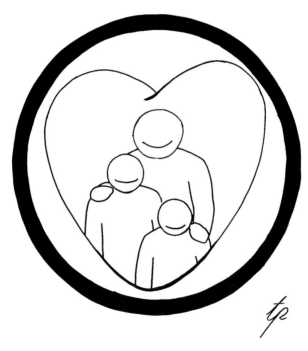

Patients and families help identify what we are doing well and also they can help pinpoint areas that may need improvement. Patient and families' advisors can provide:

- Insights about the health care providers' strengths and areas where changes may be required
- Feedback on practices and policies that those who use our services find meaningful and useful in helping them be active partners in their care
- Timely feedback and a fuller picture of the care experience than standard patient satisfaction surveys can provide.

Over to you staff nurse

Think of the various ways in which patients and their families can provide you with feedback on the care you have provided as well as the care and the services that other members of your organisation have provided.

Charmel and Frampton (2008) have identified the longer term benefits when engaging the patient and family:

- Enhanced health outcomes for patients
- Reduced errors and adverse events
- Increased patient involvement
- Reduced risk of malpractice/misconduct
- Increased employee satisfaction
- Improved financial performance.

The Royal College of Physicians (2013) note that in order for partnership working to become a reality this partnership working must be woven into the fabric of health care at every level – policy, planning, organisational and individual.

The NHS Constitution

The core principles of the NHS are applied across the United Kingdom. When the NHS was created it was founded on a number of sound principles whereby good health care would be available to all, regardless of wealth. It was based on three core principles:

- That it meet the needs of everyone
- That it be free at the point of delivery
- That it be based on clinical need, and not ability to pay.

The NHS Constitution (DH, 2013) lays down the principles and values of the NHS in England; the devolved administrations in Northern Ireland, Wales and Scotland are responsible for developing health policies of their own. The principles promoted in the Constitution apply to all patients, not only those receiving care in the hospital setting.

The Constitution sets out rights to which patients, public and also staff are entitled and pledges which the NHS is committed to accomplish, together with responsibilities, which the public, patients and staff owe to one another; this aims to ensure that the NHS operates in a fair and effective way. The law requires the Secretary of State for Health, all NHS bodies, the private and voluntary sectors who provide or supply NHS services and local authorities in the exercise of their public health functions to take account of this Constitution when they make their decisions and when they act.

Over to you staff nurse

The NHS Constitution is required to be revised every 10 years. If you were charged with contributing to its review, is there anything in the current Constitution that you would leave in take out, or is there anything you would want to add?

The seven guiding principles

There are seven guiding principles detailed in the Constitution that guide all that the NHS does:

1 The NHS provides a comprehensive service, available to all based on individual needs respecting people's human rights irrespective of gender, race, disability, age, sexual orientation, religion, belief, gender reassignment, pregnancy and maternity or marital or civil partnership status. The service diagnoses, treats and improves both physical and mental health. As well as this, it has a wider social duty to promote equality with respect to groups or sections of society where improvements in health and life expectancy are not keeping pace with the rest of the population.

2 Access to NHS services is based on clinical need, and not an individual's ability to pay. Services are free of charge, except in limited circumstances sanctioned by Parliament.

3 The NHS aspires to the highest standards of excellence and professionalism in the provision of high-quality care that is safe and effective, focusing on patient experience; it does this through the people it employs and in the support, education, training and development they receive; in the leadership and management of its organisations; and through its commitment to innovation and to the promotion, conduct and use of research. Respect, dignity, compassion and care should be at the core of how patients and staff are treated.

4 The NHS aspires to put patients at the heart of everything it does. It supports individuals to promote and manage their own health. Services reflect

the individual needs and preferences of patients, their families and their carers; they will be involved in and consulted on all decisions about their care and treatment.

5 The NHS works across organisational boundaries and in partnership with other organisations in the interest of patients, local communities and the wider population. The NHS is an integrated system of organisations and services bound together by the principles and values reflected in the Constitution.

6 The NHS is committed to providing best value for taxpayers' money and the most effective, fair and sustainable use of finite resources. Public funds for health care will be devoted solely to the benefit of the people that the NHS serves.

7 The NHS is accountable to the public, communities and patients that it serves. The NHS is a national service funded through national taxation, and it is the Government which sets the framework for the NHS and which is accountable to Parliament for its operation. The system of responsibility and accountability for taking decisions should be transparent and clear to the public, patients and staff.

Figure 6.1 illustrates the seven guiding principles and how they are all inextricably linked.

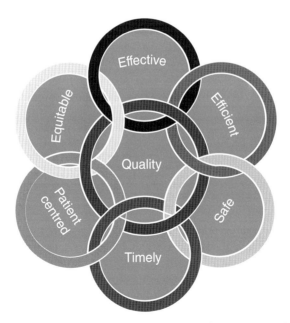

Figure 6.1 The seven interlinked principles associated with the NHS Constitution.

Table 6.1 The values that underpin the NHS Constitution.

Working together for patients	Patients come first in all that we do. The needs of patients and communities come before organisational boundaries. When things go wrong we speak up
Respect and dignity	We value every person, patient, their families or carers, or staff – as an individual, respect their aspirations and commitments in life, and seek to understand their priorities, needs, abilities and limits. We take what others have to say seriously. We are honest and open about our point of view and what we can and cannot do
Commitment to quality of care	We earn the trust placed in us by insisting on quality and striving to get the basics of quality of care – safety, effectiveness and patient experience – right every time. Feedback from patients, families, carers, staff and the public is welcomed; this is used to improve the care we provide and build on our successes
Compassion	Compassion is central to the care we provide; we respond with humanity and kindness to each person's pain, distress, anxiety or need. We give comfort and relieve suffering. We find time for patients, their families and carers, as well as those we work alongside
Improving lives	We strive to improve health and well-being and people's experiences of the NHS. We cherish excellence and professionalism wherever we find it – in the everyday things that make people's lives better as much as in clinical practice, service improvements and innovation
Everyone counts	Our resources are maximised for the benefit of the whole community; we make sure nobody is excluded, discriminated against or left behind

Source: Adapted from Department of Health (2013).

As well as the guiding principles there are values, pledges and rights that are applied to patients and staff. Table 6.1 outlines the values that underpin the Constitution.

Every user of the NHS has the right to seek redress or to have any complaint that they make about NHS services acknowledged within three working days and to have it investigated (DH, 2013).

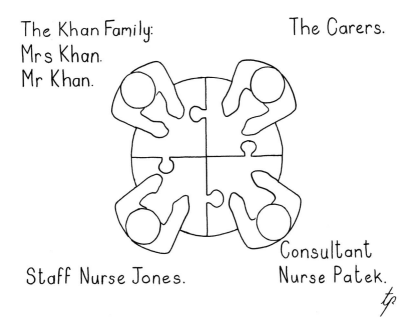

The Khan Family:
Mrs Khan.
Mr Khan.

The Carers.

Staff Nurse Jones.

Consultant
Nurse Patek.

The NHS complaints procedure

Understanding how the NHS complaints procedure works can help you help those people who may be seeking any form of redress. This can be a complex and complicated procedure for people to have to go through.

People have the right to discuss the manner in which their complaint is to be handled; they should be kept informed of progress and to know the outcome of any investigation and be provided with an explanation of the conclusions and confirmation of any action needed as a result of the complaint.

Over to you staff nurse

Undertake a review of the ways in which complaints are managed in the organisation where you work. Note where in the complaints procedure you might be involved and what might be required of you as a registered nurse.

The person making a complaint can take his or her complaint to the independent Parliamentary and Health Service Ombudsman or Local Government Ombudsman if he or she is not satisfied with the way the complaint has been managed by the NHS.

A person can make a claim for judicial review if they think that they have been directly affected by an unlawful act or decision of an NHS body or local authority. Compensation should be paid where negligent treatment has resulted in harm.

Things to consider

Complaints, their source, their handling and their outcome provide an insight into the effectiveness of an organisation's ability to uphold both the fundamental standards and the culture of caring. They are a source of information that has hitherto been undervalued as a source of accountability and a basis for improvement. Learning from complaints must be effectively identified, disseminated and implemented, and it must be made known to the complainant and the public, subject to suitable anonymisation.

The Stationery Office (2013) 'The Francis Report'

If a person is receiving an NHS service from any provider, these include
* A hospital
* GP
* Dentist
* Optician
* Community service
* NHS pharmacy
* Ambulance service or paramedic

and if that person is dissatisfied with the treatment received, he or she can speak to the service directly and talk about his or her concerns.

A person can raise concerns or pursue a complaint on behalf of someone else who is dissatisfied with treatment he or she has received or is receiving. This can be with the help of the patient advice and liaison service (PALS) or through PALS.

It may be that the person does not want to talk to the service; they may feel uncomfortable raising concerns directly, or it may be that he or she might not be satisfied with the response received. In this case, they may decide to make a complaint. A copy of the complaints procedure explaining what needs to be done or 'contact us' details can be requested.

The complaint can be raised with someone directly or by writing or emailing them. This is called local resolution.

The complaint should be made as soon as possible; this way the service can take steps to put things right immediately. If it is not possible to make the complaint right away, it must be done within 12 months of the incident or event, or 12 months from the date that the person first became aware of it.

If a person has chosen to talk to someone about his or her concerns, he or she should document the conversation, keeping it for the records. A copy of the discussion should be sent to the person for the records. An acknowledgement from the NHS service should be received within three working days. If the complaint is sent in, the 3 days start from the day that the service has received it.

If an investigation is required, this is usually concluded within 20 days and if it is likely to take longer than this, the person should be informed. A formal response will be made after the investigation.

A self-help pack is available if the person makes the complaint himself or herself. This provides all the information the person needs to make a complaint to the NHS service.

If the person is not happy with the results of the complaint, he or she can continue to work on the issue with the NHS service concerned reaching a resolution that the person finds favourable.

If however, they remain dissatisfied, the complaint can be taken to the Parliamentary and Health Service Ombudsman who will investigate the complaint and if possible will work to put things right and share lessons learned to improve NHS services.

Things to consider

People and their families are not out to complain, things happen that make them complain. I always try to listen, to stop what I am doing and give that person, their family my undivided attention, I try not to argue or interrupt. I want that person to know that I am taking his or her concern seriously. Always I empathise, I say things like 'I'm sorry that … ', or 'I understand that … '. It is important to gain as much information as I can about the problem; this helps me decide the best way to handle the complaint. Then when I have all the facts I can act.

Samira Charge Nurse

Figure 6.2 outlines the ways in which concerns and complaints can be raised.

Statement writing

The Code of Professional Conduct (NMC, 2015) requires the nurse to cooperate with internal and external investigations. As a registered nurse you may be

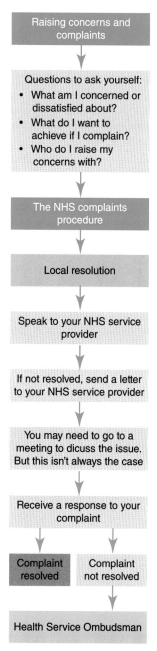

Figure 6.2 Raising concerns or complaints.   Source: Adapted from NHS Complaints Advocacy (2013).

asked to produce a statement, for a number of reasons; one reason for writing a statement may be associated with complaints. There are different types of statements, and as such you will need to consider what the statement is for and what needs to be included in it. UNISON (ND) notes that as a health worker there are a variety of reasons why you are asked to write a witness statement; writing a witness statement they suggest can be an unnerving experience. It is not unusual for some people to be frightened or worried about writing a statement.

A statement may be a written report that concerns a patient, or it may be written as a request for a professional opinion of an incident. A statement may also be requested from a witness or someone who has been involved in an incident that is being investigated. The various types of statements will have specific purposes and effects. A police statement, for example, could result in giving evidence in criminal proceedings or in a coroner's court. A statement that is made under caution could later be used in criminal proceedings as evidence. No one can be forced to make a statement if this might criminally implicate them (Royal College of Nursing (RCN), 2013a).

Over to you staff nurse

Who is your local coroner?
Where is the nearest coroner's court?
What is the role of Her Majesty's coroner?

The statement

A witness statement sets out what a witness can remember; it is a document that records the evidence of a person, which is signed by that person to confirm that the contents of the statement are true (Health and Safety Executive, 2014).

As a registered nurse you may be asked to make a statement as an independent bystander, for example, if you have witnessed a road traffic collision. You could also be asked to make a statement as a witness to an incident that you have not been directly involved in. This might, for example, include witnessing the bullying of a member of staff or a patient who is alleged to have been assaulted by a colleague (table 6.2 outlines some reasons why a statement may be required). This might lead to formal proceedings against another person where you may be required to attend a disciplinary or grievance hearing.

Table 6.2 Statements can be required for a number of reasons.

- If a patient makes a complaint. Employers must always investigate complaints and as part of this process, you and other members of staff that may have been involved in the patient's care may be asked to write a statement. This will enable the employer to collect information and address any concerns that have been raised by the patient. Every employer should have a policy for managing patient complaints
- If a patient, service user or resident has sustained an injury, his or her condition has seriously deteriorated or if something unpredicted has occurred this may be called a Serious Untoward Incident. Staff involved in the care may be required to write a statement
- If you or other members of staff are part of an investigatory procedure. If you or colleagues take out a grievance or if an investigation proceeds to a disciplinary hearing
- If there is a legal case – then the statement would be a statement required for a coroner's report or court case

Source: Adapted from UNISON (ND).

The purpose of the witness statement is to provide support to either party during an investigation/disciplinary hearing. The nurse should remember that a witness statement is a legal document and as such this can be used as evidence during these hearings and any subsequent hearings. In a witness statement, the person writing this must always provide a truthful and accurate account of the event.

Writing the statement

Preparing and writing a statement requires that you put a lot of thought into it, and put time and consideration into it to ensure that the final version is accurate, clear, concise and relevant. Be clear about what is required of you and ensure that you have all the necessary information and resources available.

Prior to writing a statement regardless of the reason you are being asked to write it, the nurse should always seek advice. This may be from a more senior member of staff or a professional organisation/trade union representative. Ensure that prior to submitting the statement they read it.

Regardless of the circumstances, a witness statement is a legal document. When it is written it must be legible and easy for anyone to read. You should always keep copies of any statements and put them away in a safe place. You may decide to send a copy to your professional organisation/trade union representative.

To reiterate, a witness statement is a legal document and as such you must always tell the truth. Be sure to give a truthful and accurate account of the event that has taken place.

Statements should reflect and relate to factual information; therefore, they should be about what was seen and what took place (not what you thought took place). They are not about speculation or what somebody else told you happened or what it was that they saw.

If you have been asked to write a statement about a person who has been in your care, you can always make a request to see the notes or documents to remind you of any involvement that you had. When writing a statement, however, you have to discriminate between the facts written in the notes and documents and what you remember – your own recollections.

Give yourself time to write the statement; do not rush this important activity. You may have been told that the statement is needed within a specific time period. You should remember that this is your statement and you should take time to ensure that you are satisfied with the content and accuracy. Nobody should change your statement without your permission.

Statement format and layout

The statement should be structured so that those reading it can work their way around it in an easy way. There is no specific structure – your employer may have their own structure/template; the following can be used as guidance.

- Number all pages.
- There should be clear wide margins on either side of each page.
- The document should be double spaced.
- Paragraphs must be sequentially numbered, short, precise and no more than six lines long.
- Where appropriate paragraphs should have subject headings.
- Write in the first person (i.e. I, me).
- The statement should be typed. If this cannot be done then use plain white A4 paper, writing neatly in black ink or ballpoint (remember this may be photocopied).

On the front page, enter:

- Your full name
- Your occupation or job title
- Your professional address
- Subject of statement (e.g. who it is about, the incident and where it was alleged to have taken place, i.e. location).

The introduction

The introduction should say who you are, your professional qualifications and when you gained them, how long you have been in your current role, your grade and your experience (each point should be a new paragraph).

The narrative (the body of the statement)

- This should be presented in a chronological order explaining the event, incident or accident
- Use subheadings and new paragraphs to structure your statement, for example:
  - Response to allegations
  - Informal meetings held
  - Telephone calls made.

Summary

When summarising or making your closing statement, recap the main points and do not add any new information or comments at this point.

Statement of truth

At the end of the statement you should make a statement of truth:
- 'This statement is true to the best of my knowledge and belief'
- Name
- Your signature and title
- Date.

References and appendices

Make a list of all documents referenced in your statement including:
- Patient records, notes and ward/departmental documents
- Any pertinent local policies or procedures
- Any relevant national standards or evidenced-based information
- Professional codes and guides.
  Once the statement has been written, check the content for:
- Accuracy
- Relevance
- Clarity – avoid generalisations, if you are using abbreviations then write the subject of an abbreviation or acronym in full the first time it is mentioned
- Concise – adhere to the points raised but, do not sacrifice essential detail for the sake of brevity. Follow a logical sequence
- Clear language – any intelligent layperson should be able to understand the content
- Compliance – follow any professional codes, local policies and confidentiality guidelines.

Nursing and Midwifery Council's investigations

The NMC exists to protect the health and well-being of the public and provides standards and rules for practice; it also investigates allegations made against nurses who are alleged to have failed to have adhered to and followed the tenets enshrined within the Code.

When the NMC receives an allegation about a nurse an assessment of the allegation is made by the NMC's Screening Team prior to making a judgement as to whether this should be referred to the NMC's Investigating Committee for a decision. When the Screening Team is carrying out its assessment, they decide if there is an allegation of impaired fitness to practise and if this is within the NMC's jurisdiction, that is, if it is in the form required by their legislation and the NMC (2013).

If a decision is made to proceed with the matter then a full investigation into the allegation is undertaken in order for the Investigating Committee to make an informed decision as to whether there is a case to answer and where necessary, the Conduct and Competence Committee or Health Committee can make a final decision on what to do.

Employers, colleagues, patients and members of the public can raise allegations concerning a nurse's fitness to practise. Referrals to the NMC must be made in writing and at this point the nurse has an opportunity to comment.

When a nurse receives a notice of a referral from the NMC it can have a devastating effect on the nurse who receives it. Disbelief, shock and anxiety are common emotions (Catterall, 2013). The nurse who has been referred to the NMC will be told that an investigation is being carried out into his or her practice and conduct and a case officer managing the case who he or she can contact at any time is allocated to him or her. The role of the case officer will be to keep the nurse up to date and to answer any questions about the process.

If a panel decides that there is no case to answer then the case is closed. If it has been decided that there is a case to answer, this is referred, for example, to the Conduct and Competence Committee or the Health Committee for adjudication. Adjudication refers to the panel process of deciding whether an allegation is proved; if it is proven, the action or sanction to be imposed is agreed. Panels may adjudicate cases at meetings; here they work purely on the paperwork collected for the case, or there may be hearings when they can hear evidence from those concerned in person. It is here where witness statements may be taken, called for and taken into account.

When a Conduct and Competence Committee or a Health Committee panel determines an allegation of impairment proved, they can choose from a range of actions or sanctions depending on the severity of the case.

Table 6.3 An aide-mémoire for statement writing.

- Be completely honest and state if you cannot remember something
- Avoid ambiguity or any subjective statements
- Avoid opinion or speculation; state facts only
- Avoid abbreviations or jargon
- Explain why you made the decisions you did or took a particular form of action
- State clinical guidelines at the time of the incident (sometimes you will be asked to provide a statement of your involvement in an incident that may go back several years); attach the relevant guideline if it is appropriate
- Retain a copy of the statement for yourself
- Seek advice from a senior member of staff or professional organisation/trade union representative
- Do not sign any statement if you disagree with the content

It is essential therefore that any statement written is clear and unambiguous and that it is honest and objective; this can help employers and regulatory bodies such as the NMC to make informed decisions in a fair, transparent, robust and timely manner. See table 6.3 for an aide-mémoire regarding statement writing.

Resources

There are a number of resources available to help nurses write statements and to support them through processes that may require them to attend a hearing as a witness to provide evidence. Legal advice and assistance may need to be considered; a professional organisation/trade union may (but not always) be able to provide this advice (RCN, 2013b).

Voluntary organisations such as the Citizens Advice Bureau and independent advisors can also be used a resource.

Conclusion

Patients, those who provided care and governments all agree that involving patients in health care decisions is the right thing to do. It must be acknowledged that this will take time and above all commitment by all parties to make this a reality.

Making investments in shared decision making will help build a high-quality health care system. It will mean that those who provide care as well as patients will need to take on new roles and delivery systems. Teams and technology will need to be developed in order to develop these new roles. When nurses, health care organisations and patients work together, they will make use of the best medical evidence ensuring that patients get the best care possible. Patients deserve to have the knowledge and skills to make wiser health care decisions, and nurses have the skills to provide them with this knowledge and equip them with the skills needed. Health care organisations can deliver better care to all patients when they also have the tools, training and support in place to communicate effectively. Shared decision making is key to creating a health care system that values patients as partners and delivers truly patient-centred care.

One aspect of providing safe and effective nursing care is to listen to the compliments and the complaints people make about us. The NHS complaints procedure can be complex; when possible complaints made should be dealt with using local resolution. The nurse may be required to provide a statement (e.g. a witness statement) and if this is needed then there are processes and structures in place to help the nurse do this in an effective manner.

References

Berwick, D.M. (1997) "Medical Associations: Guilds or Leaders". British Medical Journal, Vol 314, No **7094**, pp. 1564–1565.

Catterall, L. (2013) "Called to an NMC Hearing". Practice Nursing, Vol 24, No **3**, pp. 149.

Charmel, P.A., Frampton, S.B. (2008) "Building the Business Case for Patient-centered Care". Healthcare Financial Management, Vol 62, No **3**, pp. 80–85.

Department of Health (2013) "The NHS Constitution. The NHS belongs To Us All" http://www.nhs.uk/choiceintheNHS/Rightsandpledges/NHSConstitution/Documents/2013/the-nhs-constitution-for-england-2013.pdf last (accessed January 2015).

Health and Safety Executive (2014) "Witness Statements" http://www.hse.gov.uk/enforce/enforcementguide/investigation/witness-witness.htm last (accessed January 2015).

National Health Service (2013) "How to Make A Complaint About an NHS Service" http://nhscomplaintsadvocacy.org/what-is-nhs-complaints-advocacy/how-to-make-a-complaint-about-an-nhs-service/ last (accessed January 2015).

Nursing and Midwifery Council (2013) "Witness Information. Investigations". NMC: London.

Nursing and Midwifery Council (2015) "The Code, Professional Standards of Practice and Behaviour for Nurses and Midwives" http://www.nmc-uk.org/Documents/NMC-Publications/NMC-Code-A5-FINAL.pdf last (accessed January 2015).

Royal College of Nursing (2013a) "Statement Writing" http://www.rcn.org.uk/_data/assets/pdf_file/0012/489495/Statement_writing_-_Advice_guide_Final_V3_2.pdf last (accessed January 2015).

Royal College of Nursing (2013b) "On the Case: Advice Support and Representation from the RCN". RCN: London.

Royal College of Physicians (2013) "Royal College of Physicians, Position Statement: Personalising Healthcare: The Role of Shared Decision Making and Support for Self-Management" https://www.rcplondon.ac.uk/sites/default/files/rcp_position_statement_on_shared_decision_making_and_support_for_self_management.pdf last (accessed January 2015).

The Stationery Office (2013) "The Francis Report. The Report of the Mid Staffordshire NHS Foundation Trist Public Inquiry" http://www.midstaffspublicinquiry.com last (accessed January 2015).

UNISON (ND) "Guidance on How to Write a Witness Statement" http://www.swamb.com/graphics/cms/HC-60-11%20How%20to%20write%20a%20statement%20attachment.pdf last (accessed January 2015).

CHAPTER 7

New ways of working: advancing nursing practice

Aim

This chapter aims to provide insight into the many roles that nurses are undertaking in order to advance nursing practice and enhance the patient experience.

Objectives

By the end of this chapter you will be able to:

1 Describe the concept of advance practitioner
2 Outline key features of the role
3 Discuss the role and function of the advanced nurse practitioner
4 Consider the advantages of undertaking an advanced nursing role
5 Highlight the professional development opportunities associated with this role
6 Describe the role and function of the nurse prescriber

Introduction

The health and social care landscape continues to change at a pace in order to meet the health and social needs and demands of the population, a different population profile to that at the time the NHS was first formed. The nursing and other health care professions have responded to these changes, taking the lead in challenging established professional boundaries.

The Essential Guide to Becoming a Staff Nurse, First Edition. Ian Peate.
© 2016 John Wiley & Sons, Ltd. Published 2016 by John Wiley & Sons, Ltd.

New ways of working are about creating and sustaining a capable, flexible workforce in order to respond to the needs of people who use health and social care services in a safe, effective and efficient way. Advancing practice and developing new ways of working bring with them opportunities and challenges. With the introduction of new roles this means that nurses are still required to take on responsibility for the care and the advice that they offer the people they provide care to (DH, 2010a).

Workforce planning undertaken by health care organisations has to ensure that the skill profile of the team can match the needs of the people they serve and in so doing this is in alignment with the Health and Social Care Act 2012, whereby the patient was to be at the heart of all that is done (see also the NHS Constitution (DH, 2013)). As a result of this opportunities have been and continue to be taken to develop nurses into enhanced or extended roles; however, this can only be effectively achieved with appropriate education, training and support. At all times, the nurse must only ever take on an extended role if this is in the best interests of the patient.

Accountability and responsibility

Those nurses who take on advanced roles are accountable to different authorities for the discharge of their responsibilities, in several ways. This discharge of duty is central to accountability and is central to the role of the advanced practitioner.

Employee responsibilities are defined by a contract of employment and usually include a job description that sets out responsibilities in detail. These objectives should be discussed, developed and clarified with the nurse's manager informally and formally, usually as a part of the performance appraisal process that should be held at least annually. It is important that the nurse understands the link between their work objectives, those of the team, those of the organisation and most importantly those of the people he or she serves (see figure 7.1).

Professional responsibilities are defined by a duty of care to those who use nursing services and the Code of Professional Conduct. Nurses are required to recognise and observe the limits of their training and competence and satisfy themselves that anyone else to whom they refer is also appropriately qualified and competent (NMC, 2015).

Legal responsibility (as defined by Statute and in common law) is a part of professional responsibility and describes the obligation to comply with the law. There are elements of stature evident within guidance and standards issued by the NMC.

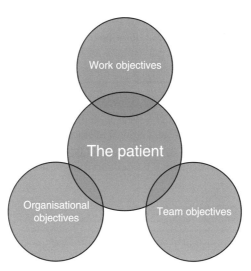

Figure 7.1 Inter-relationships associated with the role of the advanced nurse practitioner.

Over to you staff nurse

Go to the NMC web site www.nmc.org.uk and make a list of the guidance and the standards that the NMC produce.

Standards and guidance

There are many organisations and institutions that issue standards and guidance, for example, the Royal College of Nursing's guidance; the Nursing and Midwifery Council also issues guidance as well as standards. The National Institute for Health and Care and Excellence (NICE) and the Scottish Intercollegiate Guidelines Network (SIGN) provide clinical guidance. There are important distinctions between guidance and standards.

Standards

The Nursing and Midwifery Order 2001 requires the NMC to establish standards of proficiency that have to be met by applicants wishing to be admitted to the various parts of the register. These standards are deemed essential for the delivery of safe and effective practice and are set out within the standards for each part of the register (nursing, midwifery and community public health nursing) and for recordable qualifications such as nurse prescriber. The important point about standards is that they have the full authority of the law.

Guidance

Again, the Nursing and Midwifery Order 2001 requires the NMC to provide and publish guidance that reflects what it considers is best practice. There is some flexibility in how guidance is applied to practice. Where it is not followed precisely, then the nurse will be called to account for this and may have to explain how an alternate approach can or has produced a similar outcome.

From novice to expert

Benner (1984) suggests that in the acquisition and development of a skill, a nurse passes through five levels of proficiency: novice, advanced beginner, competent, proficient and expert (see figure 7.2).

In table 7.1 Benner's stages of clinical competence have been outlined.

At the end of the nurse's 3-year education programme the NMC (2010) requires that the nurse has been deemed competent to practice. This is assessed theoretically and practically.

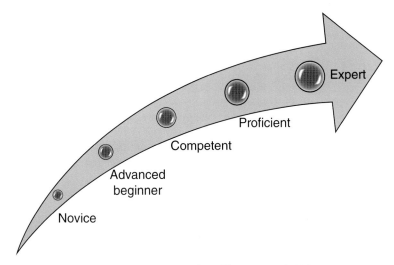

Figure 7.2 From novice to expert. Source: Adapted from Benner (1984).

Table 7.1 Stages of clinical competence.

Novice:

The novice or beginner has no experience in the situations in which he or she is expected to perform. The novice lacks confidence to demonstrate safe practice and requires continual verbal and physical cues. Practice is within a prolonged time period and he or she is unable to use discretionary judgement

Advanced beginner:

Demonstrates marginally acceptable performance because the nurse has had prior experience in actual situations. He or she is efficient and skilful in parts of the practice area, requiring occasional supportive cues. May/may not be within a delayed time period. Knowledge is developing

Competent:

The nurse who has been on the job in the same or similar situations for 2 or 3 years can be deemed competent. The nurse is able to demonstrate efficiency, is coordinated and has confidence in his or her actions. For the competent nurse, a plan establishes a perspective, and the plan is based on considerable conscious, abstract, analytic contemplation of the problem. The conscious, deliberate planning that is characteristic of this skill level helps achieve efficiency and organisation. Care is completed within a suitable time frame without supporting cues

Proficient:

The proficient nurse perceives situations as whole rather than in terms of chopped up parts or aspects. Proficient nurses understand a situation as a whole because they perceive its meaning in terms of long-term goals. The proficient nurse learns from experience what typical events to expect in a given situation and how plans need to be modified in response to these events. The proficient nurse can now recognise when the expected normal picture does not materialise. This holistic understanding improves the proficient nurse's decision making; it becomes less laboured because the nurse now has a perspective on which of the many existing attributes and aspects in the present situation are the important ones

Expert:

The nurse who is considered expert has an intuitive grasp of each situation and zones in on the accurate region of the problem without wasteful consideration of a large range of unfruitful, alternative diagnoses and solutions. The expert nurse operates from a deep understanding of the total situation. This nurse's performance becomes fluid and flexible and highly proficient. Highly skilled analytic ability is necessary for those situations with which the nurse has had no previous experience

Source: Adapted from Benner (1984) and Jasper and Mooney (2013).

Things to think about

How has your role changed since you became a registered nurse? How do you know that you are competent to practice?

Competent nurses

These nurses are able to demonstrate that they are aware of patterns of patient responses and are able to draw on past experiences; they have developed their technical skills and they use policies and procedures to inform any current situations that they are faced with; they are accountable and responsible for their practice. The competent nurse working as a member of the multidisciplinary team is fully aware of his or her role and contribution within the team as well as understanding the limitations of his or her own practice.

Competent nurses start on their journey of incrementally building on their knowledge and skills development and they are aware of their own learning and evolution as practitioners. Competent nurses are confident in what they know, their skills repertoire and their ability to provide safe and effective patient care. These nurses make up most of the nursing workforce.

Proficient nurse

Benner (1984) describes a proficient nurse as one who has an in-depth knowledge of nursing practice that is a result of the time and experience that they have amassed in a specific clinical area. These nurses depend on previous experience to guide their decision-making and problem-solving. This is different from the competent practitioner who has relied more on the explicit use of rules and theoretical perspectives to inform his or her practice. Knowledge and experience are integrated into a whole at the proficient stage and sources of information are drawn upon in an intuitive way (Jasper and Mooney, 2013).

Paradigm cases have been described by Benner (1984), which enables the practitioners to adapt to any unplanned events enabling them to respond with speed, efficiency, flexibility and confidence as these nurses do not have to stop to consciously work out and think about the course of action. The proficient nurse sees patients in a holistic way as individuals providing an integrated, collaborative approach to care in order to ensure that the most suitable package of care is formulated and provided. Standards of practice are used only as guidelines, and decisions are made on the basis of evidence-based practice using the best available evidence that is merged with clinical judgement; this slows these practitioners to modify treatment regimens that will meet individual patient need.

These practitioners assume a leadership role within the clinical practice area; they act as a role model, preceptor and coach and act as a resource for others in the profession. Practice is characterised by higher level cognitive skills, as they are able to predict patterns and outcomes, critically analysing clinical situations and seeking alternative courses of action. These practitioners are usually employed in a care management role, for example, ward or clinical nurse manager, or they may undertake a specialist role after years of experience in the speciality.

Proficiency follows competency as a result of experience and development within that particular area (Benner, 1984).

Expert nurse

Expert nurses carry out their work from an intuitive base – they develop a comprehensive knowledge base through years of experience that is associated with continuous professional development. The expert practitioner can therefore function independently, being self-directed, flexible and innovative when providing patient care. Experts are reflective practitioners who function from a deep understanding of a total situation with the aim of resolving complex issues when not all of the salient information is present; they are critical thinkers. While performing as an independent practitioner, the expert also works in a collaborative manner with the interprofessional team, ensuring that the patient is at the centre of all that is done.

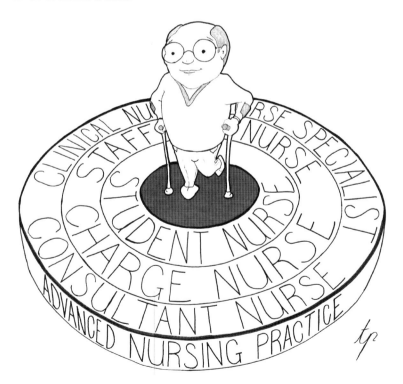

Expert nurses act as change agents, moving practice forward and contributing to the knowledge base in their sphere of expertise. The role of the consultant nurse (an expert practitioner) (Department of Health, 1999) is made up of four core components:

1 Expert practice
2 Professional leadership and consultancy
3 Education and development
4 Practice and service development.

Consultant nurses are considered to be at the leading and cutting edge of their speciality as well as retaining a clinical component of their role as they continue to practise their speciality.

Mullen et al. (2011) suggests that nurse consultants lead, drive and support quality improvement, increase productivity and service effectiveness. Sturdy (2004) also suggested that these nurses are taking forward a variety of important service improvements and initiatives, as they undertake postgraduate study.

Advanced nurse practitioner

Nurses continue to extend and expand their scope of practice beyond their initial registration (first level) in all care settings. Nurses now work at advanced practice level in areas such as general practice and community health, acute care, hospice settings, sexual health, aesthetic nursing and mental health.

The title advanced nurse practitioner has led to much consternation. There are nurses who use the title nurse practitioner or advanced nurse practitioner and some of these have not undertaken the educational preparation that is required to work safely at an advanced level.

There have been concerns regarding the existence of the plethora of job titles that are being used; they suggest that this does not help the public to understand the level of care that they can expect. There are nurses who have job titles that would appear to imply an advanced level of knowledge and competence; however, some of these nurses may not have such knowledge or competence. As these nurses often act as independent practitioners, their practice may not be subject to the scrutiny of another professional and as such what they do may not be subject to governance.

The DH (2010b) notes that the term 'advanced level practice' has been applied inconsistently to a number of different roles and that this can often lead to confusion about the scope and competence required for this level of practice.

To reiterate, all registered nurses are bound by *The Code* (NMC, 2015) and this includes those who are practicing at an advanced level. The following assumptions apply:

- All registered nurses take personal responsibility for their actions and omissions; they fully recognise their personal accountability.
- All registered nurses are able to make sound decisions about their continuing personal and professional development; they practise within the scope of their personal professional competence and extend this scope as appropriate; delegating aspects of care to others and accepting responsibility and accountability for such delegation; and working harmoniously and effectively with patients and their carers, families and friends and colleagues.
- All registered nurses are expected to conduct themselves and practise within an ethical framework that is based upon respect for the well-being and safety of those they provide care to.

The European Working Time Directive introduced in 1993 has meant that nurses are undertaking treatment and care that was once firmly located within the domain of other health care professionals, particularly doctors. Advanced nursing practice has been actively promoted since the 1980s with the intention of enhancing service delivery and improving the health outcomes of diverse patient groups. This is done through the development of competences and accreditation (RCN, 2012a) and has provided a solid foundation for current and ongoing developments.

The RCN, the UK Modernising Nursing Careers initiative (DH, 2006) and in alignment with the UK, European and international literature, defines advanced nursing practice as a level of practice as opposed to a role or job title. Advanced nursing practice builds on, and supplements, those competencies that are common to all registered nurses.

In an elaboration of the definition provided by the DH (2010b) they recognise that there are two levels of nursing practice: the first relates to first level registration (entry into the profession) and the other is at advanced level. Advanced level is where the registered nurses are working at a level that is well beyond initial registration, and they use existing knowledge and skills to support and further develop their practice. Specific tasks according to the DH (2010b) do not define advanced level practice; tasks that were once considered to be extended role activities, for example, intravenous drug administration and cannulation, are now, following appropriate preparation, the expected skills base required of all registered nurses who practise in areas where these are essential elements of nursing practice.

Advanced level practice includes aspects of education, research and management; however, it is resolutely grounded in the provision of direct care or clinical work with patients, families and communities. Those nurses who opt to work at an advanced level promote public health and well-being. They have an understanding of the implications of the social, economic and political context of health care. The advanced nurse practitioner's expertise, experience and professional and clinical judgement are shown in the expert nature of their practice and the wisdom of their knowledge. The advanced nurse practitioner's expertise, experience and professional and clinical judgement have been highly developed and this is acknowledged and recognised by others (such as patients and other professionals); they possess extensive knowledge in areas such as diagnostics, therapeutics, the biological, social and epidemiological sciences and pharmacology and their enhanced skills in aspects such as consultation and clinical decision-making. Those who work at an advanced level apply complex reasoning, critical thinking, reflection and analysis that inform their assessments, clinical judgements and decisions, applying knowledge and skills to a wide range of clinically and professionally challenging and complex circumstances.

Nurses working at advanced level are autonomous, self-directed, manage their own workload, and work across professional, organisational, agency and system boundaries aiming to enhance services and develop practice – they act as practice leaders. They undertake, assess and manage risk and proactively challenge others about risk. Advanced practitioners network locally, regionally, nationally and internationally, developing productive relationships with a number of stakeholders in order to shape the strategic direction of services for the benefit of those who use them.

The advanced nurse practitioner is constantly working to improve the quality of services and patient care using a range of data, tools and techniques to improve practice and health outcomes, demonstrating their impact and value.

Those who work at an advanced level are at the forefront of their sphere of practice, identifying their own and others' personal and professional development needs, taking effective action to address them.

The advanced nurse practitioner is likely to have a track record of innovative practice and service development, such as taking a lead in designing and delivering new care pathways and services and in the development and implementation of policy, standards, guidelines and protocols.

The RCN (2012a) suggests that advanced nursing practice provides new opportunities for nurses with regard to career pathways and professional development. The RCN, the NMC and the health departments of the countries of the United Kingdom strive to identify and implement appropriate strategies that will help realise enhanced patient safety and public protection.

All nurses who are advancing nursing practice are regulated by the NMC's Code (NMC, 2015); however, this may not be sufficient when used in isolation and other checks and controls must be in place (RCN, 2012a). Improving employer-led governance is another key component of the wider framework and employers should produce guidance that enables the monitoring of advanced nurse practitioners and as such can ensure improved patient safety. The use of local governance frameworks can assist in assuring fitness for practice and as a result public protection. Robust governance activity by employers makes clear the advanced nurse practitioner's responsibility for patient safety; it also provides an additional level of monitoring of appropriate competency, education and the application of evidence-based practice.

Over to you staff nurse

Think of your own area of practice and the organisation in which you work identify those who hold the title of advanced nurse practitioner or nurse practitioner. What is their role and function, how were they prepared for this role and how does their job differ from that of any other senior nurse?

Becoming an advanced nurse practitioner

Those wishing to become an advanced nurse practitioner should undertake an appropriate accredited advanced nursing practice programme (RCN, 2102a). The programme should include core areas that build upon the nursing skills that the nurse has already acquired. The programme is theory and practice based (the RCN (2012a) suggests 50% theory and 50% practice) and the aspiring advanced practitioner must achieve a set number of competencies. It is usual for the employer and the institution providing the programme to require a number of years post registration experience in a senior position prior to commencing the course. Table 7.2 provides a list of subject areas that may be included.

The advanced nurse practitioner role is usually offered at master' level; however, there has been no consensus regarding this. The RCN (2012a) suggests that the level of practice within which advanced nurse practitioners work encompasses the following:

• Making professionally autonomous decisions
• Receiving patients with undifferentiated and undiagnosed problems and undertaking an assessment of their health care needs, based on highly developed nursing knowledge and skills that are not usually exercised by nurses, such as physical examination
• Screening patients for disease risk factors and early signs of illness
• Making differential diagnoses

Table 7.2 Some subject areas that are usually included in a programme of study designed for advanced nurse practitioner.

- Therapeutic nursing care
- Comprehensive physical assessment of all body systems across the life span
- History-taking and clinical decision-making skills
- Health and disease, including a holistic approach that encompasses the physical, sociological, psychological and cultural aspects of the person and the family
- Applied pharmacology and evidence-based prescribing
- Management of patient care
- Public health and health promotion
- Research and evidence based practice
- Organisational, interpersonal and communication skills
- Accountability – including legal and ethical issues
- Quality assurance and governance
- Political, social and economic influences on health and social care
- Leadership and teaching skills

Source: Royal College of Nursing (2012a) and Department of Health (2007).

- Developing with the patient an ongoing nursing care plan for health, emphasising health education and preventative measures
- Requesting appropriate investigations and providing treatment and care individually, as part of a team and through referral to other agencies
- Providing a supportive role in assisting people to manage and live with illness
- Having the authority to admit or discharge patients from their caseload and making appropriate referrals to other health care providers
- Working in a collaborative manner with other health care professionals and disciplines
- Offering a leadership and consultancy function as needed.

Over to you staff nurse

Make a list of the pros and cons of being a nurse practitioner.

Pros	Cons

Table 7.3 Some assessment strategies that may be used in programmes offered to potential advanced nurse practitioners.

- A personal and professional portfolio
- Written examination(s) (can include multiple-choice questions)
- Submission of written assessments
- A collection of case studies
- Objective structured clinical examination(s)
- Poster presentations
- Viva voce
- Assessment undertaken in the work place (facilitator feedback)

Assessment of the programme is rigorous and is carried out at several appropriate stages. Assessment is designed to determine that the programme's learning objectives/outcomes have been met and at the appropriate academic level. Table 7.3 discusses a number of assessment strategies that can be used.

Professional indemnity

Commencing 17 July, 2014, the UK government introduced a new requirement for all health care professionals to have in place suitable indemnity arrangements. The law requires that nurses have in place an appropriate indemnity arrangement if they are to practise and provide care. The arrangement does not need to be held by an individual nurse; however, it is the nurse's responsibility to ensure that he or she has appropriate cover. If a nurse practises without indemnity cover he or she will be breaking the law.

Most nurses will already meet the requirement and will not need to take any further action. Nurses meet the requirements where:

- They work exclusively for the NHS
- They work in an employed environment in the independent sector where the nurses' employer provides them with indemnity cover
- They undertake self-employed work and have made their own professional indemnity arrangements.

If a nurse is self-employed then he or she will need to arrange his or her own cover. This may be as part of a membership of a professional body or trade union, directly from a commercial provider or this may be a combination (NMC, 2014).

As nurses are responsible for maintaining their registration with the NMC, when the nurses first register or renew their registration, a number of self-declarations confirming that they meet the standards for registration will need to be signed. These declarations now include holding appropriate indemnity insurance.

Nurse prescribing

Nurse prescribing in the United Kingdom has grown significantly over the last decade; a number of key stakeholders have an interest in nurse prescribing, such as, the Department of Health, the NMC and the RCN. Significant legislative and policy reforms have been required to make nurse prescribing a reality; this has encouraged and supported nurses to take on prescribing roles in the acute and community setting. It was the Cumberlege Report in 1986 that first recommended that community nurses prescribe from a restricted list of drugs and applications; the publication of this report was the momentum that was required to begin this long and arduous journey. Gradually, nurses were granted prescribing powers; district nurses and health visitors first gained access to a limited national formulary in 1998 and progression with nurse prescribing continued very slowly (RCN, 2012b). Objections for progression initially came from medical health professionals; these declined as evidence emerged with regards to the improvements made in access, patient safety and patient-centred care. These continue to bolster the foundations supporting nurse prescribing.

Things to consider

What are the legal, professional and ethical issues that nurses must think about prior to agreeing to take on an extended role?

The primary legislation that allows nurses to prescribe is the Medicinal Products: Prescription by Nurses and Others Act 1992. Chapter 28, Article 1(d) of this act defines a nurse prescriber as 'any registered nurse, midwife or health visitor'. Under the legislation prescribers have to have sufficient knowledge and competence to:

- Assess a patient/client's clinical condition
- Undertake a thorough history, including medical history and medication history, and diagnose where necessary, including over-the-counter medicines and complementary therapies
- Decide on management of presenting condition and whether to prescribe or not
- Identify appropriate products if medication is required

- Advise the patient/client on effects and risks
- Prescribe if the patient/client agrees
- Monitor response to medication and lifestyle advice.

Non-medical prescribing

Non-medical prescribing is the prescribing of medicines, dressings and appliances by health professionals who are not doctors. There are two types of nurse prescribers (RCN, 2012b):

1 Nurse independent prescribers: these are specially trained nurses who are allowed to prescribe any licensed and unlicensed drugs within their clinical competence. Nurse prescribers were given full access to the British National Formulary (BNF) in 2006, giving nurses parity with doctors concerning prescribing capabilities. Since April 2012 nurse independent prescribers have been able to prescribe controlled drugs within their competence.

Community practitioner nurse prescribers are a different group under independent prescribers. These nurses consist of district nurses, health visitors and school nurses who are allowed to independently prescribe from a limited formulary known as the Nursing Formulary for Community Practitioners, which includes over-the-counter drugs, wound dressings and applications.

2 Nurse supplementary prescribing is based on a voluntary prescribing partnership between a doctor (independent prescriber) and a nurse (supplementary prescriber) where the supplementary nurse prescriber has the ability to prescribe any drug listed in a patient-specific clinical management plan after the patient has been diagnosed by a doctor. There are no legal restrictions on the clinical conditions where the supplementary prescriber cannot prescribe and this is most beneficial for those nurses caring for patients with long-term conditions such as diabetes and asthma.

Patients have reported a high level of satisfaction and confidence in nurse prescribing. Jones et al. (2011) have demonstrated that effectiveness of nurse prescribing in acute care settings found no difference in prescribing methods between nurses and doctors in hospitals; however, nurse prescribing helped patients though better use of available skills set on the wards and increased reports of patient satisfaction. Patients are able to access clear information and advice on disease progression and can clarify questions they have on medication side effects, dosage calibration and when to administer medicines with nurse prescribers, ensuring correct medication use and concordance. Furthermore, the incidence of medication errors by nurse prescribers is minimal (Jones et al., 2011; Stenner et al., 2011).

In the United Kingdom the benefits of nurse prescribing have been constantly reported. These reports show enhanced patient care and satisfaction, better access to medicines, reduction in waiting times and delivery of high-quality care (RCN, 2012b).

Nurse prescribing brings with it a number of benefits for patients, the organisation in which the nurse works as well as for the nurse. Patients will be able to access the right medicines they need at the right time, from the right person. This can result in avoiding delay in receiving medicines, a fall in the number of unnecessary appointments with various health professionals, a reduction in the risk of hospitalisation and quicker recovery. Patients will also be provided with more choice with regard to who it is that they choose to see concerning their health care.

For the organisation, there is a better use of the workforce; there are financial savings in terms of less appointments needed, less inpatient costs and possibly faster recovery. There is a more efficient delivery of service for patients and professionals.

For the practitioner, there is raised professional self-esteem in being able to provide a whole package of care for patients. Staff who are motivated are ideally placed to be innovative in their approach to service delivery.

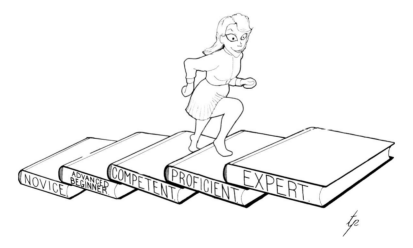

Conclusion

Nurses are continually striving to advance their practice with the key aim of ensuring that the patient is central to all that is done. They do this by ensuring that their practice is up to date and evidence based. New ways of working have allowed nurses to venture into fields of practice that had hitherto been in the domain of other health care professionals, such as doctors.

Competent nurses are the main stay of the NHS. Through further professional development and knowledge and skills acquisition nurses can become proficient and an expert practitioner taking on the multifaceted and complex role of advanced practitioner.

References

Benner, P. (1984) "From Novice to Expert: Excellence and Power in Clinical Nursing Practice". Addison-Wesley: Menlo Park.

Department of Health (1999) "Making a Difference: Strengthening the Nursing, Midwifery and Health Visiting Contribution to Health Care". HMSO: London.

Department of Health (2006) "Modernising Nursing Careers. Setting the Direction" http://www.dhsspsni.gov.uk/modernising_nursing_careers-2.pdf last (accessed January 2015).

Department of Health (2010a) "Responsibility and Accountability Best Practice Guide – Moving on From New Ways of Working to a Creative, Capable Workforce". DH: London.

Department of Health (2010b) "Advanced Level Nursing: A Position Statement" https://www.gov.uk/government/uploads/system/uploads/attachment_data/file/215935/dh_121738.pdf last (accessed January 2015).

Department of Health (2013) "The NHS Constitution. The NHS belongs To Us All" http://www.nhs.uk/choiccinthcNHS/Rightsandpledges/NHSConstitution/Documents/2013/the-nhs-constitution-for-england-2013.pdf last (accessed January 2015).

Jasper, M. and Mooney, G. (2013) "The Context of Professional Development" in Jasper, M., Rosser, M. and Mooney, G. (Eds) "Professional Development, Reflection and Decision-Making in Nursing and Health Care", Ch 1, pp. 6–40. Wiley: Oxford.

Jones, K., Edwards, M. and While, A. (2011) "Nurse Prescribing Roles in Acute Care: An Evaluative Case Study". Journal of Advanced Nursing, Vol 67, No 1, pp. 117–126.

Mullen, C., Gavin-Daley, A., Kilgannon, H. and Swift, J. (2011) "Nurse Consultants 10 Years on: An Insight to the Role for Nurse Managers". Journal of Nursing Management, Vol 19, pp. 820–831.

Nursing and Midwifery Council (2010) "Standards for Pre registration Nursing Education" http://standards.nmc-uk.org/PreRegNursing/statutory/background/Pages/introduction.aspx last (accessed September 2015).

Nursing and Midwifery Council (2014) "Professional Indemnity Arrangement. A New Requirement for Registration" http://www.nmc-uk.org/Documents/Registration/PII/PII%20final%20guidance.pdf last (accessed January 2015).

Nursing and Midwifery Council (2015) "The Code. Professional Standards of Practice and Behaviour for Nurses and Midwives" http://www.nmc-uk.org/Documents/NMC-Publications/NMC-Code-A5-FINAL.pdf last (accessed January 2015).

Royal College of Nursing (2012a) "Advanced Nurse Practitioners. An RCN Guide to Advanced Nursing Practice, Advanced Nurse Practitioners and Programme Accreditation". RCN: London.

Royal College of Nursing (2012b) "RCN Fact Sheet. Nursing Prescribing in the UK". RCN: London.

Stenner, K., Courtenay, M. and Carey, N. (2011) "Consultation Between Nurse Prescribers and Patients with Diabetes in Primary Care: A Qualitative Study of Patient Views". International Journal of Nursing Studies, Vol 48, No 1, pp. 37–46.

Sturdy, D. (2004) "Consultant Nurses: Changing the Future". Age and Ageing, Vol 33, pp. 327–328.

CHAPTER 8

Becoming a manager

Aim

The aim of this chapter is to introduce and build upon the readers' understanding of the concept of management in order to enhance their management skills.

Objectives

By the end of this chapter you will be able to:
1 Distinguish between management and leadership
2 List the characteristics of an effective manager and leader who influences
3 Consider the concepts power and authority
4 Discuss the change process
5 Describe team working

Introduction

In your new role you will realise that you are expected to act as a manager and you will be required to delegate to other staff, some of whom may not be registered nurses. It is likely that you will have to blend clinical and business management skills. Just as it may be a challenge to transition into being an effective clinician the same can be said of being an effective manager. With time and commitment, both clinical and managerial skills will develop. Management is something that you will need to give much consideration to.

You will be expected to deal with patient safety concerns, quality improvement projects, staff (and their issues), finance and budgeting and many other tough issues. While all of this may not be required when you first start your job there

---

The Essential Guide to Becoming a Staff Nurse, First Edition. Ian Peate.
© 2016 John Wiley & Sons, Ltd. Published 2016 by John Wiley & Sons, Ltd.

will be an expectation that as your skills (clinical and otherwise) develop you will assume more and more management responsibilities, which will include delegating to others. Remember that Rome was not built in a day.

Some of the issues that you will need to give consideration to when you become a manager are highlighted in table 8.1.

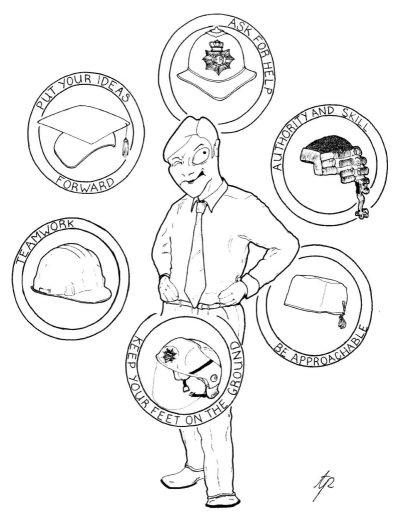

Spencer et al. (2014) note that when you move from being a staff nurse to sister/charge nurse (another transitional phase in your career) there will also be a number of issues that you will need to take into consideration. Some of

Table 8.1 Becoming a manager.

- Keep your feet firmly on the ground
- Plan and prioritise the work you have to do
- Always be realistic concerning what can and cannot be achieved
- Ask for help
- Have a mentor/clinical supervisor/preceptor
- Go over and revise your objectives
- Appreciate the priorities and pressures of others
- Work closely with the charge nurse
- Undertake appropriate delegation
- Be proactive and put your ideas forward
- Challenge but do this in the best interests of your patients
- Give and be prepared to receive feedback
- Be approachable
- Understand you cannot do everything at once
- Be confident and say no when appropriate
- Remember that you do make a difference

Source: Adapted from Spencer et al. (2014).

these issues become even more apparent when transitioning from student to staff nurse, such as being self-aware, managing yourself, managing time and adapting to change.

Things to think about

Employee rights

Employers have to respect a wide range of employee rights. These include providing employees with a healthy and safe working environment, allowing them to belong to a trade union and providing pay statements.

Can you think of any other employee rights that as a manager you must be aware of?

The staff nurse as manager

One aspect of the newly qualified staff nurse's job description will relate to management. The staff nurse will be required to manage human and material resources and the job description may also refer to managing self as in managing stress. Figure 8.1 provides an overview of a job description and the expectations of a band 5 staff nurse.

THE ROYAL HOSPITAL NHS TRUST JOB DESCRIPTION
Registered Nurse Band 5

Key Working Relationships:
All members of the nursing team, medical staff and other professionals allied to medicine.

Job Summary:

1 To work in accordance with the NMC's Code of Professional Conduct and relevant professional guidelines as a named nurse or key worker (with facilitation) for a distinct group of patients and to take responsibility for
   ◦ the assessment of care and health education needs
   ◦ the development, implementation and evaluation of packages of care including discharge planning for each patient.
2 To gain experience and skills in
   ◦ clinical practice
   ◦ mentioning, facilitation and teaching
   ◦ management (as appropriate).
3 To work in accordance with the Royal Hospital Strategy for nursing and to contribute towards achieving its objectives
4 To maintain effective communication
5 To participate in clinical supervision as appropriate and to teach and act as a facilitator/mentor/preceptor/role model to less experienced members of staff.

1 **Patient Care Responsibilities**
   1.1 Acting as a Named Nurse, to maintain accountability for assessing, planning, implementing and evaluating packages of care within the framework of team nursing
   1.2 To co-ordinate the patient's discharge
   1.3 To promote a patient-focused approach to care working with all relevant health professionals
   1.4 To provide education to patients and their carers as required
   1.5 To provide information which enables patients to make choices about adopting a more healthy lifestyle
   1.6 To complete patient documentation correctly
   1.7 To maintain a safe environment
   1.8 To contribute to the establishment and monitoring of protocols/care pathways
   1.9 To participate in the promotion of effective communication
   1.10 To ensure patient confidentiality.

2 **Professional Development and Education Responsibilities**
   2.1 To develop own teaching skills and take part in staff/student education programmes
   2.2 To help maintain a suitable learning environment for staff and act as a facilitator in the supervision and teaching of less experienced staff
   2.3 To attend orientation programmes and mandatory training sessions
   2.4 To be responsible for developing and sustaining own knowledge, clinical skills and professional awareness in accordance with PREP requirements and to maintain a professional portfolio with evidence of reflective practice

Figure 8.1 A standard band 5 staff nurse's job description. Source: Adapted from Spencer et al. (2014).

2.5 To contribute to annual appraisal and be responsible for own personal and professional development

2.6 To contribute to a programme of clinical supervision

2.7 To assist in the development and implementation of nursing practice guidelines, standards, policies and procedures

2.8 To assist in the training and development of health care assistants and complete assessors training as required.

3 **Research and Development Responsibilities**

3.1 To assist in promoting nursing practice aligned to relevant research

3.2 To maintain an awareness of evidence-based practice

3.3 To contribute to research and development programmes within the ward.

4 **Audit, Quality and Risk Management Responsibilities**

4.1 To take part in the setting and monitoring of measurable standards of care and be accountable for maintaining standards

4.2 To maintain understanding of the national, professional and local quality issues appropriate to the delivery of nursing services

4.3 To uphold quality initiatives that enhance 'customer care' and promote relationships between staff, patients and visitors

4.4 To participate in the audit activity for monitoring and reviewing nursing quality

4.5 To be aware of personal responsibilities concerning the maintenance of a safe environment and identification of potential risks for all staff, patients and visitors, taking action as and when required

4.6 To be aware of the role of the nurse in handling complaints in accordance with policy

4.7 To participate in maintaining a clean environment

4.8 To recognise own training needs, to ensure individual is informed and competent in the use of all equipment provided for use.

5 **Resource Management Responsibilities**

5.1 To develop and maintain an understanding of budgeting, exercising care and economy in the ordering and use of equipment

5.2 To assist in the assessment and monitoring of staffing requirements and report difficulties to the appropriate manager.

Figure 8.1 (*continued*)

Over to you staff nurse

In the job description provided in figure 8.1 dissect out the various roles of the staff nurse and pay attention to the professional aspects of the job, clinical attributes associated with the job, the educational aspects and the managerial elements.

Leadership and management

Leadership and management go hand in hand. They must go hand in hand but they are not the same thing; they are distinct but complementary. The word 'leadership' comes from words of Anglo Saxon and Nordic origin that mean 'route', 'path' and 'journey' and as such leadership is concerned with 'direction' and 'movement'. 'Management' comes from the Latin word 'manus', which means 'hand', so management is about being 'hands-on'. Henri Fayol defined management as planning, organising, commanding, coordinating and controlling the work of a given set of employees (Wren, 1972). See table 8.2 for a comparison of the two concepts.

Comparing and contrasting the practices of management and leadership can help clarify the unique features of these activities (Swanwick and McKimm, 2011b). The terms are often used interchangeably; however, Wilcox (2014) suggests that a leader selects and takes on the role whereas a manager is appointed or is assigned to take on the role. Managers are responsible for ensuring that organisational goals are met and that staff undertake organisational tasks; they manage much of the day to day activity on the ward. Another attribute that is associated with the manager is that of directing; this is where the manager has to tell staff what to do. The manager has to choose the right type of communication in this instance; this is all dependent on the situation (context). There are some situations that may call for announcement only – a directive approach that requires direct action and other situations that invite input from staff; it is always more preferable to seek input from others where possible.

Table 8.2 Management and leadership.

Management	Leadership
• A science	• An art
• Granted, given	• Earned
• Speed oriented	• Direction oriented
• Coordination	• End back planning
• Resource and logistically oriented	• People oriented
• Day to day	• Visionary
• Reactive	• Proactive
• Relies on authority	• Charismatic
• Doing things right	• Doing the right thing
• Relies on rank	• Mental resilience
• Manipulates/conducts	• Care oriented
• Sets instructions	• Sets example

Source: Adapted from Mullins (2013), Wilcox (2014) and Swanwick and McKimm (2011a).

Make a list of situations you are facing or that you may face that require you as the manager to seek input from others or where you might have to take a more directive approach, where you require some form of direct action.

Seeking input	Directional

In a leadership role the leader influences others. It is of course desirable that managers are good leaders; however, there are leaders who are not managers and there are also some managers who are not leaders.

Mullins (2013) suggests that management takes place within a structured organisational setting and with prescribed roles; it is focused on the attainment of aims and objectives. Management is achieved through the efforts of other people. When people manage they make use of systems and procedures. Leadership is principally associated with getting others to follow, or encouraging others to do things willingly. It is concerned with a relationship through which one person influences the behaviour or the actions of other people. Leadership does not necessarily occur within a structured environment. Bennis and Nanos (2007) suggest that leaders are people who do the right thing and managers are people who do things right. An effective leader will inspire people.

Take some time and think about people who you would say are good leaders.

What made you think this?

Managing people can be a challenge because humans can be wilful and unpredictable (and this includes you); they have different interests and objectives. As well as this, organisations (internal and external to the NHS) face constantly changing circumstances.

Skills required to manage effectively

Self-awareness

One of the greatest skills required to manage effectively is your ability to be self-aware. Self-awareness involves closing the gap between the nurse's own perception of self and the perception others have of him or her. Self-awareness is more than asking 'Who am I?' For the nurse it is more important to ask 'What effect, at this moment, am I having on other people?' Having a firm understanding and acceptance of his or her own self will allow the nurse to recognise differences and uniqueness in patients.

It is not always easy to confront or accept some aspects of ourselves; this can be painful. However, identifying what our strengths are and working on our weaknesses and becoming self-aware has the potential to lead to a positive self-concept, which can in turn increase our self-esteem and so enable us to increase this same quality in others.

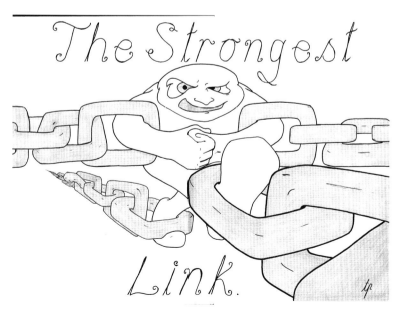

Self-awareness does not occur as a one-off activity, it is a process or continuum. There are several methods the nurse can use to achieve self-awareness; they may include self-initiated activities, for example, reflective practice and self-assessment; more formal processes can occur through appraisal, 360° feedback (this usually includes direct feedback from an employee's subordinates, peers and supervisor(s), as well as a self-evaluation), mentoring and clinical supervision. Learning through reflection is a key requisite for self-awareness and can be used as a tool for lifelong learning.

There are a number of ways the nurse can undertake self-awareness exercises; these can be carried out alone, using introspection or with others in an interactive way. You are familiar with a range of reflective models where you write or talk about an event asking questions about it, such as:

- How did this happen?
- Why did the health care assistant react to me in this way?
- What lessons can be taken from this event for learning for the next time if I find myself in a similar situation?

Self-analysis can include completing exercises or tests, tests that are designed in order to identify a person's qualities, beliefs, values, strengths and weaknesses to help improve interactions with others. The tests and exercises can be completed by the person alone or as a group.

Being more self-aware and using the knowledge gained can assist us when our concerns with 'self' hinder our capacity to help others (Rowe, 1999). Transactional analysis, six-category intervention analysis and the Johari Window are key theories that can be used when considering self-awareness. You will have used at least one of these theories during your preregistration nursing programme.

Eckroth-Bucher (2010) notes that self-awareness has long been seen as fundamental for the professional nurse with the accepted view that being more self-aware can lead to greater competence, something the staff nurse constantly strives to improve upon. Self-awareness is a dynamic, transformative process of self. Self-awareness is the use of self-insights and presence knowingly with the intention of guiding behaviour that is genuine and authentic; through self-awareness therapeutic care can improve.

Time management

Time management involves the use of processes and tools in order to gain maximum efficiency, effectiveness and productivity. It requires the nurse to master a set of skills such as the setting of goals and planning and to use time effectively to achieve the desired results. Making better decisions concerning how and what is done can help enhance performance.

Getting everything done in an effective manner requires time management. The only thing you can be absolutely sure of when managing your time is that there are 24 hours in a day comprising 1440 minutes; there is no possibility that you can change this. While we cannot create more time we can manage the way in which we manage the time that we have available. Keyes (1991) coined the term timelock. Timelock is akin to gridlock where traffic becomes so congested that it can no longer move. In timelock the excessive demands being made on our time mean we simply have no time left.

You know that nursing is a demanding job and that sometimes it may feel as if there are not enough of those 1440 minutes in the day to do all the work that needs doing. Unlike other jobs the thing about nursing is that the priorities change as the patient's condition dictates (and it might have been this that you saw as an attractive factor when thinking about nursing as a career). That well-prepared to-do list may no longer be relevant as you attend to a patient whose needs are urgent.

Making time to meet personal, professional, family and organisational goals is central to your overall success as each impacts on the other. Neglecting any of the elements can be detrimental to your overall health and well-being as well as your performance as a staff nurse. Using time management hints, tips and suggestions may help you manage your time in a more effective manner, making your life a little easier and as a consequence the patient's also. Nurses need to work smarter not harder.

There are a number of resources available to managers:

- People
- Equipment
- Money
- Time.

Out of all of these, it is time that is irreplaceable, which means that time management skills are therefore the key for success according to Pearce (2007).

There will always be constant demands on your time and attention and it can be difficult to identify what your priorities are when there is so much to be done. When working with people and when providing patient care, priorities can change quickly and you need to be able to hone and develop your skills to allow you to re-assess situations and to make appropriate responses. As with making any decision, when you are establishing priorities you need to be aware of the consequences of this, for example, what will be the consequence if this is not done right away, in the next hour, during this shift and so on. There are some priories and the decisions about them that will be more evident than others; managing the safe environment of a person having seizure is more of a priority than answering a telephone.

Time is a valuable resource and not all nursing time is spent on direct patient care. Managing your time involves planning ahead and realising that unforeseen events may disrupt this plan. LEAPS is a mnemonic used by Walton and Reeves (1996) that can help in time management:

List the activities to be done
Estimate time needed to carry out each activity
Allow time for unscheduled activities or errors
Prioritise activities
Study the activities of the day.

Over to you staff nurse

As a newly registered nurse you are managing a group of six patients in a bay. The ward is busy and the phone is ringing constantly; the ward administrator is late. The Specialist Registrar has arrived for a round and asks you to accompany the team; you have a confused patient and she is wandering into other bays. At the same time, Mr Aziz has rung his nurse call bell and he is trying to attract your attention.

Thinking about the above scenario, in what order of priority would you deal with the issues?

What are the factors that have to be considered in order to make your decision?

What might be the consequences of your actions?

Being 'time challenged' is something many nurses will have experienced; there are a variety of reasons for this such as, spending too much time on mundane tasks, sifting through papers and permitting others to dictate your time.

Covey (2004) when considering the habits of highly effective people suggests prioritising activities that are urgent, non-urgent, important and not important. Using this approach can help nurses develop planning skills that permit a wider vision. This in turn can lead to the effective use of a list that will allow the nurse to have less of a focus on those activities that fall into the non-urgent category.

Time management and management of self are dependent upon each other. If the nurse manages self better then time will also be better managed. Understanding this can assist the nurses in then moving on to develop techniques to better manage their time. Time should be viewed as ever changing and can with practice become a process that can be controlled.

Controlling the situation

Nurses who are time challenged can begin to regain control with the implementation of a few basic techniques.

- Ignore the phone: Do not feel pressured to go and answer the phone every time it rings. Many phone calls are not urgent and they will only distract you.
- Prioritise: Make a list! Make a priority list that details the tasks to be completed. When you formulate the list do this in order of urgency and number them; number one will be your highest priority. The formulation of the list in itself can be a challenge all on its own, but it is an essential requirement. Depending on the time frame of your jobs/tasks, revisit the list, maybe on a weekly basis to better manage the flow of your week. Do not forget to assign time in your schedule to review your list daily and track your progress towards the completion of that project or goal; it can be very satisfying to physically cross things of the list.
- Eliminate clutter: Keep your work area clean and clutter free as well as your head; this will help you focus on the important things.
- Delegate: This skill develops over time as you become more confident in yourself and those you work with. It is a misconception by many managers that in order for a project to be completed, they have to hold the decision-making power on every level. Appropriate delegation of tasks and projects is an asset for effective time management.
- Be self-centred: Remember that your time is indeed your time. Schedule time for you to complete tasks without interruption from those around you. Being self-centred allows you to have better control of your day and create dedicated work time to complete the number one task on your priority list. It also provides downtime to process the results of decisions and to reorganise any changes to your priority list.
- Set goals: Goals are established in an attempt to motivate you towards the completion of a task. You already know that goals have to be specific, time orientated, achievable, measurable and realistic. Unrealistic goals will result in discouragement and disillusion and cause your time to dissipate.
- Say 'No': There are times when you really must say no. Constantly agreeing to do things and saying yes will only lead to stress, frustration and time wasting.

Types of power

Understanding the concept of power and how it can be used and abused when working with others can help the manager work in a more effective way. As the nurse gains experience as a staff nurse, they will develop expert power; they do

Table 8.3 Types of power.

Type of power	Brief description
Legitimate power	This type of power is connected to a position of authority as a result of the position the individual holds. The ward sister has legitimate power and authority as a result of the position held
Reward power	This is linked closely with legitimate power; it comes about because the manager has the power to provide or withhold rewards
Coercive power	Coercive power derived from the fear of consequences is associated with the threat of punishment. This type of power can also be used against staff members when, for example, there is the threat of receiving unfavourable nursing work
Expert power	Based on specialised knowledge, skills or abilities, expert power is recognised and respected by others. The individual is perceived as an expert in an area and has power in that area as a result of this expertise. For instance, the breast cancer nurse has expertise in the care of individuals who have had breast cancer. As a result of this, other nurses seek out the breast cancer nurse as a resource and use the expert's knowledge to guide the care for these patients
Referent power	This is power that a person holds because others identify closely with that person's personal characteristics; they are liked and admired by others. Individuals who have knowledge that is needed by others to function effectively in their roles have information power. A person may, for example, withhold information from others in order to maintain control. The manager who gives directions without providing needed information on rationale or constraints is abusing information power
Leadership power	This is the ability to create order from conflict, contradictions and chaos. This happens when the staff or people involved in the conflicts have a trust for that manager who is able to influence people to respond because they want to respond

Source: Adapted from Wilcox (2014) and Sullivan and Decker (2009).

this by increasing competency in their role and with their clinical skills. Wilcox (2014) notes that there are many different types of power (see table 8.3).

Honing those interpersonal skills that will improve your ability to work with others means you may need to use various types of power. These skills will include communicating what people need to know clearly and completely as you provide support to them as they work to accomplish the stated goals. You should be willing to demonstrate to others a willingness to give and receive feedback as you manage them; this is important when working to develop and enhance power in working relationships with others.

You should also be aware of what can detract from power. Some of your behaviours can cause this detraction, for example, coming across as being disorganised, in the way you present yourself or in how you work, engaging in unprofessional behaviour, such as, gossiping or being unnecessarily critical of others.

Things to think about

Harassment

In the Equality Act 2010 harassment is defined as 'unwanted conduct related to a relevant protected characteristic, which has the purpose or effect of violating an individual's dignity or creating and intimidating, hostile, degrading, humiliating or offensive environment for that individual'.

Think about this and what this might mean for you as a manager.

What does your organisation policy say about bullying and harassment?

Change management

The ongoing state of many health care organisations is one of change. The rate and complexity of this change adds to intense emotions that play out both inside and outside organisations.

There are times when change is deliberate and is a product of conscious reasoning and actions; this type of change is known as planned change. On the other hand, on occasions, change can unfold in an apparently spontaneous and unplanned way and this is known as emergent change. Nurses experience both types of change; your role is to work through the change process as well as helping others to work through it. Understanding the emotional phases of the change process highlighted in table 8.4 can help you personally and others. Holbeche (2006) suggest that change, which is unexpected, can undermine confidence and threaten sense of purpose.

The catalyst for change can arise from economic, political, technological, cultural or societal sources. Reactions to change can include fear, insecurity, uncertainty, frustration, dislike, anger, sadness, depression, guilt or distrust. Some people may experience a sense of unfairness and betrayal, which can make it difficult for managers and leaders to set direction, encourage alignment and gain commitment from those in their organisation. Table 8.4 considers some of the emotional phases that are associated with the change process.

Change and how it is managed are central elements in quality and improvement processes; it is also one of the fundamental activities associated with

Table 8.4 Emotional phases of the change process.

Phase	Characteristics	Intervention
Equilibrium	High energy; feelings of balance, peace and harmony	Explain how changes may impact on the status quo
Denial	Denies reality that change is going to occur; experiences negative changes in physical health, emotional and cognitive behaviour	Actively listen, be empathetic and use reflective communication strategies
Anger	Blames others; can exhibit envy, rage or resentment	Be assertive and assist with problem solving. Encourage to determine the source of anger
Bargaining	Efforts made to try and eliminate the change; frequently talks in such terms as 'If only'	Search for real needs and problems and explore ways to achieve outcomes through conflict management strategies and win–win negotiation skills
Chaos	Diffused energy; feelings of powerlessness and insecurity along with a sense of disorientation	Encourage time for inner reflection
Depression	Devoid of energy; nothing seems to work; sorrow, self-pity and feelings of emptiness	Encourage expression of feelings of sorrow and pain. Support staff to learn to let go
Resignation	Lack of enthusiasm as change is being accepted passively	Patiently explain again, in detail, the desired change and the rationale
Openness	Some renewal of energy and willingness to take on new roles or assignments resulting from change	Allow employees to move at own pace
Readiness	Eagerly expands energy to explore new events that are happening; reintegration of emotions and cognition	Assume a directive management style; assign tasks, provide direction
Re-emergence	Expressions of empowerment as new project ideas are initiated	Together explore questions and develop an understanding of role and identity. Staff take actions based on own decisions

Source: Adapted from Perlman and Takacs (1990), Wilcox (2014) and Bach and Ellis (2013).

managing people. Those who implement change have to take the first step of disrupting the status quo, next they have the job of moving everyone and everything involved to new ways of doing things and then finally, they have to ensure that the new practices and processes do not revert back to the former state.

Table 8.5 Some barriers associated with change.

- Lack of understanding about the change itself, no clear vision, direction or priorities set
- Absence of leadership – this is required to inspire and engage people's energies as well as to keep the change moving forward
- Lack of focus and strong project management of the change – no clear lines of accountability and responsibility
- Failure to engage others and secure buy-in of key stakeholders
- No clear process for managing endings and beginnings and co-ordination of the change process
- Issues/barriers to change are not acknowledged; this results in low engagement, poor morale and a fast return to 'the old ways'
- People are not involved in development and communication
- Failure to recognise successes or celebrate these. Those involved need to see that their effort is paying off and their contributions are valued
- Not measuring progress and learning from experiences; this is essential to sustain the change

Source: Adopted from Sullivan and Decker (2009) and Bach and Ellis (2013).

Barriers to change

It helps to understand the barriers to change (actual or potential) if change is to be successful (see table 8.5). Using this knowledge, the manager can consider which barriers and levers may be relevant to a particular problem.

Team working

The most common type of team spoken about in health care is the multidisciplinary team. A multidisciplinary team includes all the health care workers who are involved in a particular patient or a group of patients' care; this might include a number of allied health and nursing staff and doctors. On a shift to shift basis there are a number of nurses providing direct patient care and the emphasis here would be on the nursing team.

The nursing team can comprise whatever groups or levels of nurses deemed appropriate by the ward staff. It will depend on the number of beds on the ward and the level of staffing and skill mix. A team should consist of a staff member who takes on the team leader role. This would commonly be a registered nurse. Some teams will be big and some will be small; there is no limit to how the team is configured so long as the configuration meets the needs of the ward. The National Institute for Health and Care Excellence – NICE (2013) have made recommendations concerning nursing staff numbers for adult acute wards.

Nurses are required to work as team members as well as working as individuals; the job description in figure 8.1 makes much reference to team work and team working. You cannot work effectively as a team member unless you are aware of your own contribution to that team, your own strength and limitations; you also have be self aware. There are no nurses (or there should be no nurses) who work in isolation. The Code of Professional Conduct (NMC, 2015) requires nurses to work with colleagues in a cooperative manner, respecting the skills, expertise and contributions of colleagues and refer matters to them when this is appropriate. In order to work as an effective team member then it is imperative that effective communication skills are used.

The New South Wales Department of Health (2011) suggests that in simple terms a team can be defined as a group of people who are mutually dependent on one another as they strive to achieve a common goal. The team acts in an interdependently dynamic way.

Team working is a key feature of working as a nurse as nurses work in multidisciplinary teams; these teams (health and social care teams) are often fluid and dynamic; the way a team performs can have a direct impact on the health and well-being of patients. Flin et al. (2008) make the point that the size and structure of a team can influence how teams perform; this, they suggest, is also true of the internal dynamics of the team members and how the group is led.

Teamwork happens through team structures and team processes. The structure is associated with size, roles and type of hierarchy and also the accepted ways of behaving (the way things are done). When structures and processes work well teams work well, they perform and they achieve; however, when they are misaligned team cohesion can be destroyed.

Team dynamics are invisible forces that work between different people or groups in a team. They can have an impact (good or bad) on how a team behaves or performs and their effects can be complex. Team dynamics are psychological processes and can be seen most clearly in the way that the group interacts. Team dynamics requires you to consider the forces that influence team behaviour; some of these include:

- Personality styles
- Team roles
- How the team communicates, cooperates, coordinates and makes decisions
- Environmental structures
- How tools and technology are used
- Organisational culture
- Processes/methodologies/procedures.

In managing team dynamics this can be done by examining the forces involved and intervening in a constructive manner to make the effects of those forces positive, when this is possible.

Biech (2008) offers 10 key points in efforts to build a successful team (see table 8.6).

Managing conflict

It is not unusual to experience conflict at work or outside of work; appropriate systems are required to manage it; conflict is inevitable when working with others. Team members will often have different perspectives and in some instances, those differences could escalate into conflict.

When working in a nursing team, team members need to have the skills to be able to approach other members who are 'not pulling their weight'. When conflict does occur there should be a standard procedure for dealing with it.

In some instances healthy conflict can be good for a team as this can generate a positive and constructive challenge as well as organisational learning. Constructive conflict can be seen as a positive thing. When a range of different

Table 8.6 Ten key points in efforts to build a successful team.

A clear vision	• The ward nurses must have a clear vision for the future and shared values displayed and revisited frequently • Individual team goals must be agreed at the start of the shift to ensure that everyone is 'pulling in the same direction'
Roles determined	• Team member's roles are clearly defined and all team members know what their jobs are • The team will be made up of different grades of nursing and the team leader role
Open and clear communication	• Open and clear communication is an essential • Listening and providing constructive feedback are key features • Communication strategies need to be in place in order to keep the team informed, focused and moving forward. This includes handover processes, convening team meetings throughout the shift, effective report writing and up-to-date care plans
Effective decision making	• Methods for effective decision making should be discussed and established
Balanced participation	• Everyone on the team should be fully involved; participation should be encouraged
Valued diversity	• All team members are valued for the contributions that they bring to the team
Managed conflict	• A process for managing conflict should be in place as this helps ensure that problems are not 'swept under the carpet'
Positive atmosphere	• There should be a climate of trust and openness for the team to work effectively • Building trust in a team can be a challenge; this does not happen overnight and requires effort
Cooperative relationships	• When there is a sense of belonging and a willingness to make things work cooperative relationships occur
Participative leadership	• Where team leaders share the responsibility and the glory, are supportive and fair, create a climate of trust and openness and are good coaches and teachers, then participative leadership can be said to have taken place

Source: Adapted from Biech (2008).

perspectives are being discussed this can bring about innovative and resourceful outcomes to problems. Here are some tips that might help you manage team conflict:

• Be aware of tensions before they are able to escalate: conduct regular one-to-one discussions with staff to keep up to date.

- As soon as you can, talk to individuals early, establishing the reason(s) for conflict; act informally in the first instance through mediation and listen.
- Be open to resolving issues: encourage immediate resolution through discussion; this can prevent any build-up of tension.
- Stay objective: this helps staff see the facts clearly with less emotion. Try not to let conflict become personal.
- Try to understand all perspectives and establish the facts prior to making any judgement.
- Address conflict in an open way: depending on the issue, suggest adopting a team approach to resolving problems. Be sure to value all contributions equally.
- Discuss the impact the issue is having or could have; do this as a team. Encourage everyone to agree to cooperate.
- Approach staff and the issues in a positive way: ask staff what they think team success might look like, how to get it and when. This creates ownership in resolving issues without having to reveal the identity of individuals or situations.
- Be clear about roles and responsibilities: make known expectations on conduct and mutual requirements needed for working well together as a team.
- Respect and protect any confidential information; this demonstrates integrity.

As a manager you will need to understand the relationships within your team and be aware of how members of your team interact with each other in order to try and avoid resentful and negative behaviours from becoming established. Valuing the various team viewpoints to avoid conflict will mean that you will have to have clear, effective communication and well-developed management skills. If you are to support your team, you need to understand how to resolve conflict and develop a team approach to avoiding unhealthy conflict.

Conclusion

Managing a team of people requires that you are able to manage yourself in order to manage them. Your skills as a manager will develop over time and indeed you will be continually honing them as not every situation you face as a manager will be the same.

The job of a staff nurse is to manage and eventually as your career progresses you will be seen not only as a manager but also as a leader. The skills, knowledge and attitudes required to be an effective manager and leader are different but they are also complementary.

In order to manage effectively, you need to have an understanding of yourself; you need to be self-aware. Being self-aware is about closing the gap between the nurse's own perception of self and the perception that others have of her/him.

Time is a valuable resource and there will be many demands made on your time. Quickly develop your skills to manage your time; do not allow others to manage this valuable resource for you.

Understanding what power is and how to use it will help you understand the various emotions associated with this complex concept. Change can also result in a number of negative emotions. Change is a complex entity but, if you understand it and why people sometimes respond to it the way they do, it will become something you might welcome. Conflict is apparent in most things we do; there can be some positive outcomes associated with conflict; however, there can also be some destructive consequences of conflict if it is not addressed.

References

Bach, S. and Ellis, P. (2013) "Leadership, Management and Team Working in Nursing". Learning Matters: Poole.

Bennis, W. and Nanos, B. (2007) (2nd Ed) "Leaders: Strategies for Taking Charge". Harper Business Essentials: New York.

Biech, E. (2008) (2nd Ed) "The Pfeiffer Book of Successful Teambuilding Tools". Wiley: San Francisco.

Covey, S.R. (2004) "The 7 Habits of Highly Effective People: Powerful Lessons in Personal Change". Simon and Schuster: London.

Eckroth-Bucher, M. (2010) "Self-awareness: A review and Analysis of a Basic Nursing Concept". Advances in Nursing Science, Vol 33, No **4**, pp. 297–309.

Flin, R., O'Conor, P. and Crichton, M. (2008) "Safety at the Sharp End: A Guide to Non-technical Skills". Ashgate: Farnham.

Holbeche, L. (2006) "Understanding Change: Theory, Implementation and Success". Elsevier: Oxford.

Keyes, R. (1991) "Timelock: How Life Got So Hectic and What You Can Do About It". Harper Collins: New York.

Mullins, L. (2013) (10th Ed) "Management and Organisational Behaviour". FT Publishing: Harlow.

National Institute for Health and Care Excellence (2013) "Safe Staffing for Nursing in Adult Inpatient Wards in Acute Hospitals" http://www.nice.org.uk/guidance/sg1/resources/guidance-safe-staffing-for-nursing-in-adult-inpatient-wards-in-acute-hospitals-pdf last (accessed January 2015).

New South Wales Department of Health (2011) "WOW: Ways of Working in Nursing" http://www.health.nsw.gov.au/nursing/projects/Documents/wow-resource.pdf last (accessed January 2011).

Nursing and Midwifery Council (2015) "The Code. Professional Standards of Practice and Behaviour for Nurses and Midwives" http://www.nmc-uk.org/Documents/NMC-Publications/NMC-Code-A5-FINAL.pdf last (accessed January 2015).

Pearce, C. (2007) "Leadership Resources: Ten Steps to Manage Time". Nursing Management, Vol 14, No **1**, pp. 23.

Perlman, D. and Takacs, G.J. (1990) "The Ten Stages of Change". Nursing Management, Vol 21, No **4**, pp. 34.

Rowe, J. (1999) "Self-awareness: Improving Nurse–Client Interactions". Nursing Standard, Vol 14, No **8**, pp. 37–40.

Spencer, C., Al-Sadoon, T., Hemmings, L., Jackson, K. and Mulligan, P. (2014) "The Transition from Staff Nurse to Ward Leader". Nursing Times, Vol 110, No **41**, pp. 12–14.

Sullivan, E. and Decker, P. (2009) (7th Ed) "Effective Leadership and Management in Nursing". Pearson: New Jersey.

Swanwick, T. and McKimm, J. (2011a) "ABC of Clinical Leadership". Wiley: Oxford.

Swanwick, T. and McKimm, J. (2011b) "What is Clinical Leadership … and Why it is Important". Clinical Teacher, Vol 8, pp. 22–26.

Walton, J. and Reeves, M. (1996) "Management in the Acute Ward". Quay Books: London.

Wilcox, J. (2014) "Challenges of Nursing Management and Leadership" in Zerwekh, J. and Zerwekh-Garneau, A. (Eds) "Nursing Today. Transition and Trends" Ch 10, pp. 194–221. Elsevier: Missouri.

Wren, D.A. (1972) "The Evolution of Management Thought". Ronald Press: New York.

CHAPTER 9

Continuing professional and personal development

Aim

This chapter aims to offer insight and understanding of the issues associated with continuing professional and personal development.

Objectives

By the end of this chapter you will be able to:
1 Discuss the concept of continuing professional and personal development
2 Highlight the key components associated with continuing professional and personal development
3 Consider the impact revalidation will have on the profession and the individual nurse
4 Discuss appraisal and the value of this activity
5 Outline the various resources available to demonstrate that you are up to date with your practice
6 Describe the professional portfolio

Introduction

In order to renew your registration every 3 years with the Nursing and Midwifery Council (NMC) you are required to provide a signed notification of practice (NoP) form and pay your renewal of registration fee. On the NoP form you are asked to make a declaration that you have met the requirements associated with post-registration education and practice (PREP) and that you are of good health

The Essential Guide to Becoming a Staff Nurse, First Edition. Ian Peate.
© 2016 John Wiley & Sons, Ltd. Published 2016 by John Wiley & Sons, Ltd.

and good character. You are also required to pay an annual registration retention fee at the end of the first and second years of the registration period.

The NMC have considered this PREP to be inadequate. The current approach is in place to ensure that in order for nurses to remain on the register they have to meet certain standards. Currently, the NMC's attempt to achieve this through a system is known as PREP. This approach is seen as inadequate as it only requires nurses to count the number of hours that have they have spent on Continuing Professional Development (CPD) and practice. There is no measure of the quality of the learning activities undertaken and furthermore, no meaningful audit of activities. Currently, this means that the NMC only has a nurse's word that they have fulfilled the requirements of PREP and that they are safe to practise. The NMC consider revalidation as the solution to these problems. All health care professions will have to have revalidation processes in place.

Revalidation

The NMC is proposing new guidelines to be met by all registered nurses when they renew their registration to practise every 3 years. Nurses will have to provide evidence in order to demonstrate that they are up to date and fit to continue practising under this proposed revalidation system. Revalidation will be replacing PREP regulatory requirements; this system was introduced in the 1990s.

All registered nurses will need to comply with the revalidation regulations after December 2015. The urgency of the need to ensure that a system of revalidation is in place was highlighted by a number of serious care failings in high profile cases such as at the Mid Staffordshire Hospital (Royal College of Nursing (RCN), 2014). In a second public inquiry in 2013 into events at Mid Staffordshire, Sir Robert Francis was asked to look particularly at the regulatory failings which had contributed to events at Mid Staffordshire Hospital. A key recommendation in the final Francis report concerning professional regulation was to implement a system of revalidation.

Those nurses who fail to comply with these regulatory requirements will no longer be registered to practise. Six key concepts associated with revalidation are outlined in table 9.1.

The NMC's aims for revalidation (NMC, 2014) are to:
- Improve public protection
- Increase public confidence in nurses and midwives by allowing them to demonstrate that they are always fit to do their work
- Ensure nurses and midwives on the register continue to meet NMC standards
- Enable nurses and midwives to be accountable for demonstrating their continuing fitness to practise

Table 9.1 Six key concepts associated with revalidation.

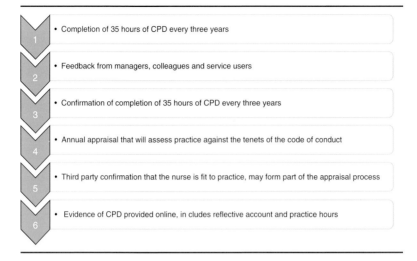

1 • Completion of 35 hours of CPD every three years

2 • Feedback from managers, colleagues and service users

3 • Confirmation of completion of 35 hours of CPD every three years

4 • Annual appraisal that will assess practice against the tenets of the code of conduct

5 • Third party confirmation that the nurse is fit to practice, may form part of the appraisal process

6 • Evidence of CPD provided online, in cludes reflective account and practice hours

- Promote a culture of professionalism and accountability through on-going reflection on the Code and Standards.

When re-registering with the NMC from January 2016 onwards, nurses will also have to re-validate and this means they have to demonstrate that they:

- Practised for the required number of hours over the previous 3 years
- Carried out learning activities that show you are complying with the NMC Code
- Collected feedback from others about your practice, reflected on it and became a better nurse as a result
- Obtained confirmation from someone well placed to comment that you remain fit to practise.

Hours of practice

The current number of hours required, which are 450 hours every 3 years, will remain. Those people who are registered as both nurses and midwives will be required to complete 900 hours.

Learning activities

There are several options available to you that will be accepted as bona fide learning. Options will include a range of CPD activities, for example, reading an appropriate professional article and completing an assignment associated with that article or reflecting on its content with regard to your practice. You will need to be able to demonstrate that the article you have read has updated your knowledge and understanding and can help you to enhance care provision.

If you undertake any in-house training at work, such as mandatory training, refresher courses or educational activities undertaken anywhere else will be considered learning. Attending a conference and writing up the experience, writing an article or presenting at a conference are acceptable examples of learning.

Over to you staff nurse

What are the 'in-house' training opportunities available in the place where you work? Do you know how to access these opportunities? Are there any prerequisites, that is, you must have been qualified for a year or more?

CPD hours

Currently, the number of CPD hours under PREP that the NMC requires each nurse to complete is a minimum of 35 hours; with revalidation this will remain a minimum of 35 hours of CPD every 3 years. The quality and the quantity of the CPD hours will be taken into account by the NMC when they carry out checks for compliance.

There are plans to stipulate that at least 20 of the 35 hours will need to be 'participatory'; what is meant by this is that the nurse will have to undertake learning with others. There are a number of ways the nurse can verify this 'participatory' learning, for example, when refreshing skills such as intermediate/advanced life support, mentoring others or participating in online discussions such as webinars.

Collecting feedback from others – (third party)

Third party feedback will need to be received, with the intention of encouraging the nurses to have reflected on their practice. It is anticipated that this feedback may come from patients, carers and in the case of educators from students or peers. This third party feedback confirms that the nurse is fit to practise. A manager, another registrant or a supervisor has to then confirm that the nurse is adhering to the Code and Standards and that he or she is fit to practise.

Third party input was chosen as user feedback is said to enhance public protection (NMC, 2014). This approach is being used by other regulated professionals such as doctors and has been further supported by a number of recent enquiries and recommendations made in the Francis Report (2013).

Table 9.2 provides you with some pointers concerning feedback.

Table 9.2 Receiving feedback.

- Ask for it
- Listen to what is being said
- Let the person who is giving you feedback finish and do not interrupt him or her – you may miss some important feedback
- Try not to rush in order to offer justification for your actions
- Ask questions to clarify anything that you do not understand
- Seek suggestions on how you might have done better
- Listen out for the good as well as the bad
- Take time to think about it – and ask other people for their feedback
- It rests with you as to whether you take action as a result of receiving feedback or not
- Think of feedback as feed forward – it can help you progress if you want it to

Appraisal

Delivering high-quality patient care is absolutely dependent on every member of staff having a clear understanding of what their role is and the part that they are expected to play in their team and organisation; staff should have an agreed set of priorities and objectives for their work. Revalidation will build on existing processes in place for appraisal. The annual appraisal will normally provide the main source of third-party confirmation and also help the nurses to reflect on their practice.

The Francis Report (2013) also made recommendations for minimum standards concerning appraisal along with the importance of professional development; the report proposed that the NMC should introduce common minimum standards for appraisal. As part of a compulsory annual performance appraisal, all nurses, regardless of where they work, will be required to demonstrate in their annual learning portfolio an up-to-date knowledge of nursing practice and its implementation. This portfolio should contain documented evidence of recognised training that the nurse has undertaken, including any wider relevant learning. There should also be evidence that demonstrates commitment, compassion and caring for patients that can be evidenced by feedback from patients and their families based on the care that the nurse has provided. The portfolio and each outcome of the annual appraisal should be made available to the NMC, should they request it as part of the nurse's revalidation activity.

Appraisal can serve a number of purposes; it provides the opportunity for a nurse and appraiser to consider the nurse's professional development over the past year and to consider developmental needs along with organisational strategic plans, for example, service developments, and to consider the skills and knowledge that the nurse will need in order to support these developments.

What appraisal is and what appraisal is not

Appraisal is …

The Scottish Executive (2004) suggests that appraisal is an activity that forms part of a continual process of planning, monitoring, assessment and support to aims, in order to assist staff to develop their skills and be more effective in their role. They add that the annual appraisal is at the heart of this process.

Appraisal is a developmental, systematic and regular review of progress that reflects on areas of strength, and where appropriate, change and improvement could be made. It looks forward to ways of preparing nurses to achieve agreed changes and reach their full potential (Health Education East Midlands, 2014).

Appraisal is a formative and developmental process, identifying individual development needs. Appraisal permits reflection on and consideration about current and future professional practice; when this is done effectively objectives and educational activities can be identified that will develop the nurse's professional and personal development.

Appraisal is not …

The appraisal process should be seen as a positive approach to development. It is not:

- About generating unrealistic expectations or rewards
- A process for evaluating/increasing pay entitlements
- A counselling exercise for non-learning and development issues
- A disciplinary procedure
- A substitute for the provision of on-going feedback to staff.

The process

There are five stages associated with the appraisal process:
- Stage 1: Preparing for the appraisal
- Stage 2: The appraisal interview
- Stage 3: Documenting the results of the interview
- Stage 4: Appraisal summary and feedback
- Stage 5: Development over the appraisal period
  The process should be viewed as a cycle and is outlined in figure 9.1.

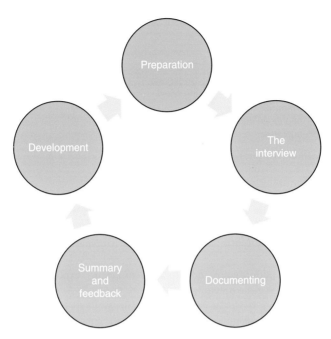

Figure 9.1 The appraisal cycle.

The stages in figure 9.1 can be adapted and tailored to meet individual and organisational needs. All stages and timings should be agreed by the appraiser and appraisee.

Price (2012) provides guidance on preparing for the annual staff appraisal. He notes that the nurse must be an active participant in the preparation for the annual appraisal interview, suggesting that preparation requires an honest and impartial self-appraisal of past work towards agreed objectives.

NHS Employers (2010) suggest that there are three phases associated with the appraisal process (see figure 9.2) – a period of preparation for the nurse being appraised and the line manager undertaking the appraisal, independently prepare for the appraisal interview … and a system whereby there is monitoring and review that occurs over the following year.

The annual process

At the beginning of the annual cycle and some weeks before the annual appraisal meeting is due, you and the manager may need to be reminded of the meeting.

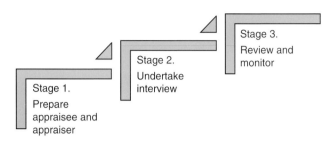

Figure 9.2 Three phase appraisal process.

Communication between both parties should detail the timetable for the meeting and the venue. Once the date has been set, you and your manager need to prepare for the meeting. In preparation consider the following:

- Reviewing current information on your job, person and skill and knowledge requirements.
- Appraise your performance and development actions, experiences and your achievements over the previous year.

You should keep a record of your achievements and experiences throughout the year. You can supplement this information with other evidence from other staff with whom you have worked. This demonstrates progression.

The meeting

The meeting is a joint responsibility and two-way discussion between you and your manager; it is expected that you will talk for much of the time, so be sure to have prepared for this. It is usual for meetings to last between 1 and 1.5 hours. If they take much longer, or far less time, this could indicate problems with the process.

The meeting opens with a confirmation of the job content/description and skill and knowledge requirements, followed by a general overview discussion of how the last 12 months have gone from a performance and development perspective. This then leads into more specific consideration of performance against objectives that have been set. Organisational objectives and values are also communicated at this point, reminding all parties of corporate objectives, relating and linking personal objectives to them. You will then be assessed against the behaviours required to be consistent with the values, as well as the knowledge and skill requirements.

A review of the past year's objectives is then undertaken, discussing your personal and work objectives agreed in the past year. You should then be encouraged to discuss your performance over the past 12 months, highlighting and describing your key achievements. Any concerns or issues you may have faced which could have held back performance and prevented any objectives being fully achieved are also considered. Your portfolio should also be referred to at this stage or at any other point in the process where appropriate.

Things to think about

Self-assessment is a tool that can help you make an analysis of your own strengths and weaknesses in the context of your annual appraisal. Some people find self-assessment difficult to undertake, despite knowing themselves and the work they do better than anyone else; the aim is to be as objective as possible. Here are some tips:

- Be proud of what you have accomplished. Emphasise the impact your accomplishments have had on you, the care you deliver and your organisation.
- Be brief. You don't have to provide a thesis; in this case, less is more.
- Be honest. Don't be tempted to inflate your ego here; being honest also includes areas where you can improve or areas that need more work.
- Be professional. This is not an opportunity for you to discuss the shortfall of your boss or the organisation. Do not be critical of others.

Over to you staff nurse

You may have been required to undertake a SWOT analysis (strengths, weaknesses, opportunities and threats) previously. Now try undertaking this in your role as a registered nurse. In this new context, new things may emerge. SWOT analysis can aid with decision making in a number of situations; it also helps you to undertake a review of where you are and where you want to be.

Strengths	Weaknesses
Opportunities	Threats

(continued)

(*continued*)

PEST analysis (political, economic, social and technological) can make you think of these external factors that can impact (positively and negatively) on your progression.

Political	Economic
Social	Technological

PESTLE (political, economic, social, technological, legal and environmental) adds two further dimensions – legal and environmental. Using this approach would make your analysis much broader.

Political	Economic
Social	Technological
Legal	Environmental

Personal and work objective setting for the next year can then proceed. This takes into account relevant organisational and departmental goals and objectives and your likely areas of work focus over the next 12 months. SMART (specific/stretching/smart, measurable, agreed/achievable, realistic/relevant and time bound) goals/objectives with clearly defined standards of achievement, and timescales should be set.

To conclude the meeting, the manager would normally summarise the discussion and actions and development plans (personal development plans) agreed and then a written summary is provided. You can then add any comments that you may have. It should be agreed when the written summary will be made available and what date the review/follow up and next appraisal will take place. A six monthly review may be the norm in the place where you work.

You should retain copies of the paperwork. You may consider putting this in your portfolio; the human resources department/your manager will also keep a copy.

Continuing professional development

CPD is a means by which members of a profession are able to maintain their knowledge and skills, developing potential in their professional lives. The concept is associated with a conscious updating of professional knowledge and the improvement of professional competence through the nurse's working life. Undertaking CPD is a legal requirement (Nursing and Midwifery Order 2001) bringing with it a commitment to being professional, keeping up to date and continuously seeking to improve. CPD is also key to updating a nurse's career opportunities.

C: Continuing – learning never stops; it is ongoing, irrespective of age or seniority; it is about lifelong learning

P: Professional – the activity focuses on professional competence

D: Development – the goal is to improve and develop the nurses' personal performance and to enhance career progression.

The NMC will be flexible around the type of CPD that you engage in; what is essential however is that you are able to demonstrate that all the activity that you undertake is related to the Code of Professional Conduct (NMC, 2015), is relevant to your sphere of practice and helps in some way to keep you up to date. This flexible approach means that your CPD can take account of how you work and where you work, for example, in direct practice, in management, education or research. This also means that you can plan your CPD activity to take account of your changing needs. The key however is to ensure that you meet the CPD requirement stipulated by the NMC.

The cost of CPD is agreed locally; for example, there are some nurses who pay for all of their own CPD activity (courses and conferences) and some employers may pay full costs or offer to support a proportion of costs.

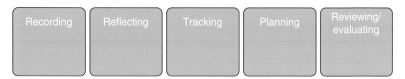

Figure 9.3 Five aspects related to CPD.

CPD refers to the activity of tracking and documenting the skills, knowledge and experience that you gain formally and informally as you work. CPD is a record of what you experience, learn and then apply to your practice; it is about leaning from your experience. The activity has to be self-directed, that is, led and driven by you. You take control of your own learning, setting your own goals and studying in the location that suits, at your own pace.

Things to consider

While self-directed learning is about you, where you take on the responsibility for your learning, it is often undertaken with others, working with your peers, as part of a network (face to face or virtual). You may come together with others for education support and peer support.

The record aspect of CPD generally refers to a physical folder or portfolio documenting development as a registered nurse. You will have been used to portfolio activity during your pre-registration nursing programme. In some cases, this can mean a training or development plan. When undertaken effectively, CPD can help you set developmental goals and objectives. CPD is a process of recording and reflecting on learning and development. There are five aspects associated with CPD; see figure 9.3.

Recording

It is up to you how you record your learning activity; there is no one set way of doing this. You may decide to keep a learning log and record your thoughts in whatever way that suits you. You may find it helpful to write things down; writing things down can compel you to think about your experiences at the time; this can make planning and reflection easier. It is not possible for you to review your experiences without recording them, even if you do have a good memory. When beginning to record your activities making responses to the following questions may help you to get started:

- Where am I now (a snap shot of your current position)?
- Where do I want to be?
- What do I have to do to get there?
- When should I review my progress?

You will need to record the steps in your professional development. These include education/training events and informal learning; you may be asked to produce this as evidence, for example, during your annual appraisal or the NMC may require you to provide this evidence to demonstrate that you are up to date.

Things to consider

Bear in mind that whenever you carry out any reflective activity, for example, writing down your thoughts, compiling your evidence, it is essential that you ensure that you maintain patient confidentiality throughout (NMC, 2015).

Reflecting

Just writing something down means that you are engaging in reflection; yet there is more to the process than just putting pen to paper. Reflecting on events and experiences helps you to integrate the learning and to determine how this might be used in other circumstances. Central to CPD is effective reflective practice. Reflective practice has the potential to help you continue with your quest to become a lifelong learner; reflective practice and reflective learning become intertwined. Your pre-registration nurse education programme has provided you with a foundation for lifelong learning. It is expected that you will continue practice as a lifelong learner (NMC, 2015).

Wigens and Heathershaw (2013) consider lifelong learning to be a process of accomplishing personal, professional, social and developmental goals throughout the individual's life span, formally and informally with the aim of enhancing individual and community lives.

Over to you staff nurse

Look again at Wigens and Heathershaw's (2013) lifelong learning definition and make a list of examples of your personal, professional, social and developmental goals and consider this retrospectively and prospectively. Have you made a difference? When you have completed this activity this will demonstrate that you are already a lifelong learner.

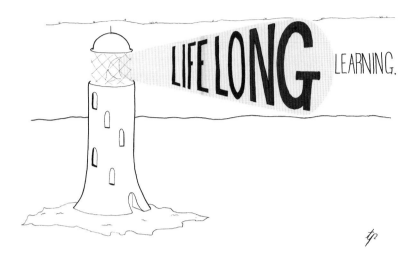

Defining reflective practice

There are a number of definitions of reflective practice; this therefore has the potential to cause confusion. Oelofsen (2012) suggests that reflective practice can be defined as the process of making sense of events, situations and actions that occur in the workplace. Roffey-Barentson and Malthouse (2009) consider 'common sense' reflection as the thoughts we have that occur during our day-to-day living, possibly after something that has occurred with a patient or colleagues that is different or challenging. These thoughts are those that we do not easily forget, maybe after a difficult encounter with a complex clinical experience or thoughts that trouble us when we feel we could do better and we try to work out how exactly. After these events have occurred we may think about the situation, thinking what went well and what did not. If the nurse reflects in this way you may be describing:

- What happened
- What you did
- What others did in response and what you did after that
- How you felt about it

This is a valuable activity where the nurse revisits and recollects the experience; he or she thinks about it, ponders and evaluates it. Working in this way, working with the experience can result in learning. After reflection comes reflective action (Polard et al., 2008) involving a willingness to engage in constant self-appraisal and development.

Crawley (2011) suggests that critical reflection is concerned with challenging and checking out what it is that you do and being prepared to act on the results. Hillier (2012) points out that when we fail to critically reflect, then what we do will remain, at best uninformed and at worst ineffective, prejudiced and constraining; in nursing this could also mean that what we do is unsafe.

The outcome of reflection may be the development of a deeper understanding of your personal skills, an enhanced self-awareness and a deeper understanding of your individual learning needs. This in turn will enhance your understanding of practice through reflection. In order to maintain your competence you must learn through practice, developing and creating your own practice.

Tracking

After you have recorded your learning, you will then be able to see how you are progressing and developing and where there are any gaps in your abilities. It is important to track progress so that you can set the direction and objectives for your future learning and training.

Planning

As in the nursing process (assess, diagnose, plan, implement and evaluate) the planning stage concerning your CPD can only take place when the previous stages have been completed.

Planning is the next step towards achieving your objectives, giving you more direction and making the activity more real as opposed to abstract. You may have noticed a gap in your abilities, for example, or when receiving feedback you might have identified room for improvement. In the planning phase you can plan direction; this may be seeking an appropriate form of education/training and going on it, attending and/or presenting at a conference, updating yourself in a specific area through reading, writing an article or just talking about it to other people.

Reviewing

Reviewing or evaluating those objectives you have set completes, and, in many ways, restarts the cycle. Personal development plans should be reviewed and revised as appropriate. You will have noticed that you have been using a systematic, as opposed to ad hoc, approach to your CPD. In this phase you can measure your progress, demonstrating that you have achieved your goals. Did you ever write that article? What about the conference you saw advertised, did you go on it?

Regularly reviewing your progress will help to keep you on track, assist with direction setting and will keep your development evolving in the way that you want it to. The evidence you amass can be used as your record of achievement.

Professional development activities

Those various activities that you undertake that have had an impact on your knowledge base, your understanding and your skills acquisition can be considered as professional development. Jasper and Mooney (2013) suggests that the most important criterion is that you can see that you are developing and changing as a result of those activities. There are formal and informal professional development activities (see table 9.3).

If you have undertaken any type of formal professional development such as a module of study (a credit bearing module) at the local university, you would have been required to undertake an assessment; this is written formal evidence. Attending mandatory training activities or a conference/seminar is a formal activity and this comes with formal evidence. Activities such as visiting a centre of excellence are less formal and in this instance the onus is on you to tailor the evidence here.

Table 9.3 Forms of professional development activities.

- Certified mandatory training
- Visits to centres of excellence
- Secondments
- Writing a protocol/guideline for your clinic
- Acquisition of an additional professional qualification
- Undertaking a systematic review of the literature
- Writing a reflective account of a critical incident
- Journal club
- Educational qualifications
- Distance learning
- Clinical audit
- Attending a conference/seminar
- Presenting at a conference/seminar
- Taking part in a webinar
- Preparing and undertaking a teaching session
- Mentoring
- Voluntary work

Over to you staff nurse

Consider those CPD activities that have been outlined in table 9.3; now allocate the activities into formal and informal.

Formal	Informal

Of course how you order these activities as formal–informal is to some extent subjective and you may find that there are some activities that straddle formal and informal.

You need to devise ways of recording your accomplishments and producing the evidence if you want this to go towards your CPD. There are a number of ways of doing this.

Storing the evidence required – the portfolio

Having amassed all of the evidence to support your CPD as well as all of the evidence you have collected during your pre-registration nursing programme and the evidence you will continue to gather as a lifelong learner, you need to store it somewhere safely and securely. The 'portfolio' is a nebulous concept as it can mean many things to many people; the portfolio should not be confused with your CV although your CV should feature in it – the portfolio does not replace the CV; it should supplement it.

McMullan et al. (2003) consider a portfolio to be a collection of evidence that is usually presented in the written form; the contents within reflect the products and processes of learning. It corroborates achievement, personal and professional

Table 9.4 The key features of a professional portfolio.

- The portfolio is personal to the individual who compiles it
- It provides a record of the individual's professional history
- It is fluid, ever changing, dynamic, reflecting the past and also projecting into the future
- It is a record reflecting particular characteristics of the person compiling
- It is made up of various types of evidence
- It is a way of critically examining how achievements have been acquired

Source: Adapted from Jasper and Rosser (2013).

development. The portfolio is merely a collection of documents presenting a picture of a practitioner transferred into words. There is no set format with regard to the portfolio but you need to give some thought to the reason you have a portfolio, who needs to access it and their reason(s).

There are advantages and disadvantages over the different types of portfolio. An electronic portfolio permits you to update it quickly; for example, when you complete your CPD activities you add this straight onto the portfolio; however, you cannot 'take' your portfolio to an interview – you will need to scan certificates of attendance if these have not be made available electronically. Electronic storage may be safer than hard copy, but losing your USB stick or loosing your hard copy portfolio is a reality using both forms of storage. Hard copy portfolios can demonstrate your personality, neat and ordered, or unattractive and disordered. Hard copy portfolios can be taken from place to place; they can, however, become bulky and at times unmanageable as well as having an impact on the environment. The key features of a professional portfolio can be found in table 9.4.

The contents of the portfolio will vary; it usually contains artefacts, tangible objects and objective documentation. Within your portfolio you may need to store the following:

- Your CV and career history
- Outstanding achievements accomplished during your pre-registration nursing programme
- Critical incident analysis
- Annual staff appraisal
- Action plans and reviews
- Person development plans
- Evidence of your CPD activity
- Appropriate certificates of attendance

Within the portfolio do not forget to record the number of hours you spend in practice and log the number of CPD hours undertaken.

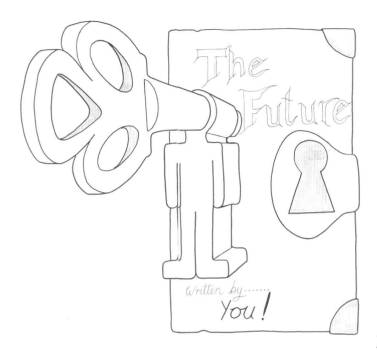

Conclusion

It is a requirement under the Nursing and Midwifery Order 2001 for registered nurses to update their professional development. Currently, these mandatory requirements are part of PREP requirements.

Providing an appropriate revalidation model that aims to ensure that the practice of nurses remains up to date is key in the quest to protect the public. The final components of the revalidation model are yet to be decided upon; however, it will have a central role to play in creating and sustaining a robust culture of professionalism among nurses.

Being able to demonstrate that you are professionally competent is a key attribute of being a registered, accountable practitioner; it is the cornerstone upon which the profession is built. All registrants are required to compile and be ready to present a professional portfolio that demonstrates their fitness to practise.

Employers are requesting nurses to present their portfolios as part of the annual appraisal process and increasingly as a component of a job application. The annual appraisal is said to feature large in the NMC's plans for revalidation.

The NMC make no specifications concerning the elements of the portfolio; it is expected that the nurse will fashion this in a way that attests the nurse's fitness to practise, containing evidence that CPD activity conforms to NMC requirements for ongoing registration.

A critical attribute of competence and CPD is your capability to learn. You need to be prepared to say that you do not know, but do not just leave it there; be committed to doing something about it.

References

Crawley, J. (2011) (2nd Ed) "In at the Deep End – A Survival Guide for Teachers in Post Compulsory Education". David Fulton: London.

Health Education East Midlands (2014) "The Practice Nurse Project. Practice Nurse Appraisal Handbook" http://www.derbyshirelmc.org.uk/pdfs/Practice%20Nurse %20Appraisal%20Handbook%20-%20FINAL.pdf last (accessed February 2015).

Hillier, Y. (2012) (3rd Ed) "Reflective Teaching in Further and Adult Education". Continuum: London.

Jasper, M. and Mooney, G. (2013) "The Context of Professional Development", in Jasper, M., Rosser, M. and Mooney, G. (Eds) (2nd Ed) "Professional Development, Reflection and Decision-Making in Nursing and Health Care", Ch 1, pp. 6–40. Wiley: Oxford.

Jasper, M. and Rosser, M. (2013) "Work-based Learning and Portfolios", in Jasper, M., Rosser, M. and Mooney, G. (Eds) (2nd Ed) "Professional Development, Reflection and Decision-Making in Nursing and Health Care", Ch 5, pp. 136–167. Wiley: Oxford.

McMullan, M., Endacott, R., Gray, M.A., Jasper, M., Miller, C.M., Scholes, J. and Webb, C. (2003) "Portfolios and Assessment of Competence: A Review of the Literature". Journal of Advanced Nursing, Vol 41, No 3, pp. 283–294.

NHS Employers (2010) "Appraisals and KSF Made Simple – A Practical Guide". NHS Employers: London.

Nursing and Midwifery Council (2014) "Revalidation" http://www.nmc-uk.org/ Documents/Revalidation/Revalidation%20factsheet.pdf last (accessed February 2015).

Nursing and Midwifery Council (2015) "The Code. Professional Standards of Practice and Behaviour for Nurses and Midwives" http://www.nmc-uk.org/Documents/NMC-Publications/NMC-Code-A5-FINAL.pdf last (accessed February 2015).

Oelofsen, N. (2012) "Developing Reflective Practice: A Guide for Health and Social Care Students and Practitioners". Lantern Publishing: Banbury.

Pollard, A., Anderson, J., Maddock, M., Swaffield, S., Wann, J. and Warwick, P. (2008) (3rd Ed) "Reflective Teaching". Continuum: London.

Price, B. (2012) "Preparing for Your Annual Staff Appraisal: Part 1". Nursing Standard, Vol 27, No 20, pp. 49–55.

Roffey-Barentson, J. and Malthouse, R. (2009) "Reflective Practice in the Lifelong Learning Sector". Learning Matters: Exeter.

Royal College of Nursing (2014) "RCN Briefing on the Nursing and Midwifery Council Consultation on a Proposed Model of Revalidation" http://www.rcn.org.uk/__data/assets/ pdf_file/0006/558519/04.14_RCN_Briefing_on_the_Nursing_and_Midwifery_Council_ consultation_on_a_proposed_model_of_revalidation.pdf last (accessed February 2015).

Scottish Executive (2004) "Framework for Nursing in General Practice" www.scotland.gov
.uk/Publications/2004/09/19966/43284 last (accessed February 2015).

Stationery Office (2013) "The Francis Report. The Report of the Mid Staffordshire NHS
Foundation Trust Public Inquiry" http://www.midstaffspublicinquiry.com last (accessed
February 2015).

Wigens, L. and Heathershaw, R. (2013) (2nd Ed) "Mentorship and Clinical Supervision Skills
in Healthcare". Cengage Learning: London.

CHAPTER 10

Teaching, learning and assessing

Aim

This chapter provides an overview of the role of the nurse in relation to teaching, learning and assessing in the practice environment. The NMC's developmental stages are described.

Objectives

By the end of this chapter you will be able to:

1 Describe the NMC's development stages of mentorship
2 Understand the responsibilities of a registered nurse in relation to teaching
3 Outline the knowledge, skills and attitudes that are essential to teach effectively
4 Discuss the opportunities that arise in care settings
5 Be aware of the challenges that the nurse may face when teaching in the clinical environment
6 Discuss the needs of the patient in relation to patient teaching

Introduction

The Code (NMC, 2015) makes clear that registered nurses have to share their skills, knowledge and experience for the benefit of people who receive care and also for their colleagues. In order to achieve this, nurses are required to:

- Offer truthful, accurate and constructive feedback to co-workers
- Deal with differences of professional opinion with other health and care professionals by discussion and informed debate, respecting their views and opinions and behaving in a professional way at all times
- Support students' and colleagues' learning to help them develop professional competence and confidence.

The Essential Guide to Becoming a Staff Nurse, First Edition. Ian Peate.
© 2016 John Wiley & Sons, Ltd. Published 2016 by John Wiley & Sons, Ltd.

It has already been emphasised throughout this book that with registration comes a change in direction in professional accountability. This brings with it wider clinical, management and teaching responsibilities; the role of the registered nurse is complex and diverse. Teaching responsibilities are concerned with developing yourself and others around you. Just as there are many theories and theorists associated with nursing practice there are also many theories and theorists related to learning and managing the learning environment along with a range of teaching strategies. There are learning opportunities in practice every day and the nurse should seize these opportunities when they arise.

Over to you staff nurse

The role of the nurse is multi-faceted and complex. Add other roles and functions to the diagram. You may need to add more spokes to the hub.

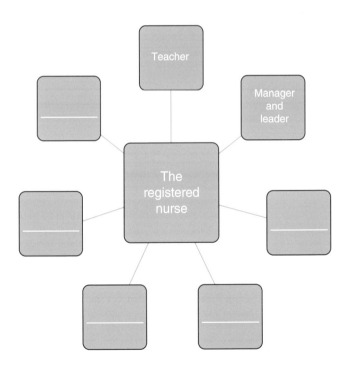

The chapter focuses on situated learning, providing the reader with insight and understanding of the key issues that are required to ensure the best use of teaching opportunities. The chapter also provides a brief discussion on the role of the mentor and the mentorship.

Standards of teaching, mentoring and assessing in practice

The NMC's standards of teaching, mentoring and assessing in practice (NMC, 2008) guide teaching and learning in practice (or situated learning) and is a key document associated with the role of the mentor. These standards provide the outcomes to be met for mentors, practice teachers and teachers and are concerned with the knowledge and skills nurses need to apply when they support and assess students in practice undertaking an NMC approved programme that leads to registration or a recordable qualification on the professional register (this is a qualification that has been approved by the NMC and can be recorded on the NMC professional register).

There are four development stages discussed by the NMC (2008) with regard to teaching, mentoring and assessing (see table 10.1).

Table 10.1 The four developmental stages.

Stage	Descriptor
I. Registered nurse	Reflects the requirements of The Code (NMC, 2015) whereby all nurses must meet the defined requirements, in particular the sharing of knowledge and support of students' and colleagues' learning to help them develop their professional competence and confidence
II. Mentor	This standard identifies the requirement for mentors. Nurses can become mentors when they have successfully achieved all of the outcomes of this stage. This qualification is recorded on the local register of mentors
III. Practice teacher	The standard here is for a practice teacher for nursing. Nurses can become practice teachers after they have successfully achieved all of the outcomes of this stage. This qualification is recorded on the local register of practice teachers
IV. Teacher	This stage is related to the standard for a teacher of nurses. Nurses can become teachers when they have successfully achieved all of the outcomes of this stage. This qualification may be recorded on the NMC register when an application to the NMC is made and the fee is paid

Source: Adapted from Nursing and Midwifery Council (2008).

The role of the stage 1 mentor

As a newly qualified nurse you are deemed a stage 1 mentor (NMC, 2008). This requires you to demonstrate your knowledge, skills and competence on an ongoing basis; you automatically assume the role of stage 1 mentor. You will be required to facilitate students and others (NMC, 2015).

You will be eligible to become a stage 2 mentor when you have successfully completed and achieved all of the outcomes associated with stage 2 mentorship, via a programme of study that is recognised by the NMC. This qualification will then be recorded on the local register of mentors that is held by the organisation where you work. In some organisations, in order to progress to a higher band, you may be required to undertake and successfully complete a mentorship pro-gramme of study. This may be offered as a standalone module or studied as part of a degree or masters programme provided at academic level 6 or 7.

The placement provider is required to hold a register of all current mentors, which includes sign-off mentors and practice teachers. Those on that register will have had to demonstrate that they have met the NMC outcomes for these roles as well as having additionally met the NMC requirements for maintenance on the register (NMC, 2008).

Kinnell and Hughes (2010) note that a stage 1 mentor begins to understand and is introduced to the roles and responsibilities of being a mentor; this can be seen as part of the stage 1 mentor's professional development. The NMC specify that a newly registered nurse cannot undergo formal preparation to become a stage 2 mentor until the nurse has been registered for a minimum of 1 year.

A stage 1 mentor is expected to support, supervise and teach students (and others). This however has to be done under the supervision of a qualified men-tor who is accountable for the student's assessment; local policies may dictate role and function. The stage 1 mentor is encouraged to contribute towards the assessment process with the stage 2 mentor, for example, in the performance of clinical skills and a contribution to the formative assessment of a student nurse.

Things to think about

The role of the stage 1 mentor

- Working as a member of a team, assisting the stage 2 mentor to mentor a student
- Working with the stage 2 mentor concerning the student's progress and needs
- A stage 1 mentor works closely with the student, providing guidance, offering counsel, demonstrating skills, making an informal assessment of competence, offering constructive feedback, encouraging reflection, acting as a role model.

(NMC, 2008, 2015)

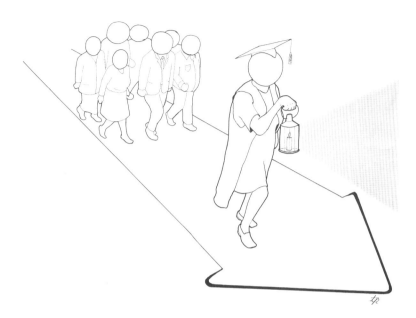

While there are many opportunities for stage 1 mentors to develop their skills in order to become stage 2 mentors, there are some activities they are unable to undertake. The stage 1 mentor cannot sign a student's practice assessment document or any document that confers student competence or undertake the final interview incorporating the ongoing record of achievement.

The NMC (2010) describe a competency as the skills and abilities required to practice safely and effectively without the need for direct supervision. Competences are achieved step by step throughout periods of practice that the student experiences during a programme of study. At the end of the final period of practice experience or supervised practice evidence of achievement is required of all competencies that will enable a sign-off mentor or practice teacher to decide if the student is deemed competent. Fitness to practice requires the student to demonstrate that they are practising safely and effectively and that they have met the standards of proficiency and all of the other requirements to become registered with the NMC.

As a stage 1 mentor you can carry out a record of orientation for the practice experience and contribute towards the continuous assessment process working in conjunction with the stage 2 mentor; the stage 2 mentor countersigns the assessment document. Without the stage 2 mentor's countersignature the assessment will be null and void. Your role is key to ensuring that the student gets as much out of the practice learning placement as possible.

Teaching and learning in the clinical setting

Teaching in the clinical environment (these can be diverse environments in different, often widely spread locations, in a range of settings in the National Health Service and elsewhere in the public, independent and voluntary sectors; NMC, 2010) is a demanding and complex task that many nurses assume without adequate preparation or orientation. Several roles have been described for those who teach in the clinical environment and these are grouped into six major tasks (Harden and Crosby, 2000):

- The information provider
- The role model
- The facilitator
- The assessor
- The curriculum and course planner
- The resource material creator.

Teaching and learning in the clinical setting takes place in a number of settings, frequently in the acute setting, in the primary care environments, in a person's home or more varied settings, for example, the prison service, hospices and others places (Wild, 2014). Wherever practice is, the learning environment can influence the quality and the experience of all patients and staff involved. Barton and Le May (2012) assert that teaching in the clinical area is one of the most important ways that the nurse learns.

The learning environment

There are many qualities or features that make an effective learning environment.

Over to you staff nurse

Make a list of what it was that you thought were the characteristics of a good learning experience when you were a student nurse; split the list up into the following (you may wish to add other bullet points):

- Environment
- Staff (include mentors)
- The manager
- Management style
- Support from the university.

Now, write a list now that you are a registered nurse.

How did you feel when you went to a new clinical environment? How can you either enhance or alleviate those feelings?

Table 10.2 Some attributes of an effective learning environment.

* Be dynamic and have democratic structures and processes in place
* A place where staff are highly valued, motivated and provide high-quality, safe and effective patient care
* Offer supportive relationships, good staff morale and a team spirit
* Have effective communication strategies in place and interpersonal relations between registered nurses and students
* Accept the student as a learner who can make a contribution to the delivery of high-quality, safe and effective patient care

Source: Adapted from An Bord Altranais (2003), Emmanuel and Pryce-Miller (2013), Wild (2014).

The purpose of clinical practice learning is to assist students to develop competence and become safe, caring, competent, knowledgeable decision-makers who are willing to accept personal and professional accountability for the evidence-based nursing care that they provide. The clinical practice experience, wherever this occurs, forms the central focus of the profession and is an essential part of the pre-registration nurse education programme. Learning in the clinical setting involves being a part of a team while learning nursing knowledge and skills. Pertinent to the practice of adult learning is the need to provide an environment of mutual respect, partnership and support along with trust.

Constructing a climate that encourages learning in complex environments can be a challenging task. The learning environment influences how the student will experience practice; positive experiences are key to learning. In table 10.2 some of the attributes of an effective learning environment are outlined.

When students feel they are part of the team, when they are offered support and encouragement they will flourish and will learn in a more effective way (Papp et al., 2003). However, when the environment is unpredictable, unstructured and overwhelming, this can lead the student to feel vulnerable and anxious. There are other issues that can threaten the student experience.

Over to you staff nurse

Think about the issues that may impact on the student learning experience, positive and negative.

Papp et al. (2003) note that issues such as staff shortages, lack of mentors, increased workload, staff that feel threatened by the student presence and poor teaching skills can add to students saying they do not feel supported.

If a positive learning environment is created, then this can provide a meaningful and safe education and development setting for all staff in the clinical setting. The purpose of a planned clinical experience can help students to improve their clinical and interpersonal skills and integrate the theory they have amassed with practice they experience. Students will also become socialised into the formal and informal roles and norms, the protocols and expectations of the profession and health care system in which they are working.

Frameworks for teaching and learning

The clinical environment is an important area for learning and nurses continue to make an enormous contribution to the education of students and others. Varieties of theories of learning available for the nurse to use are important to identify the principles of learning and understand how individual differences can impact on the learning process.

Over to you staff nurse

It is interesting to think about your own particular way of learning and to recognise that everyone does not learn the way that you do.
Find out about the different ways in which people learn.
What do you understand by the acronym VARK?

Teaching can be seen as a system of activities that have been organised to promote education or instructing. When viewed like this a deliberate and methodological activity that has within it a controlling element is a mechanistic activity. A more reflective method is suggested by Schön (1987) who emphasises a coaching approach; the learner is encouraged to seek explanations and the teacher is there to provide advice and offer clarification.

Kolb (1984) describes learning as a somewhat permanent change of behaviour, suggesting it is a 'process whereby knowledge is created through the transformation of experience'; learning becomes experiential. It is an outcome with an end-product, the change in behaviour. How learning occurs and how these processes operate is complex. It is important to remember that no one framework or no one theory can work in isolation and neither can one theory provide a full understanding of this fundamental human activity; there are many theories available to support how it is that we learn.

Table 10.3 Operant conditioning and conditional response.

Operant conditioning	Conditioned response
Original experimental work involved rats and pigeons and then later, humans. Skinner found that rats and pigeons when placed in a box containing a food tray and a lever to operate the release of the food, over time would learn the connection between pressing the lever and releasing the food	Pavlov, in his work, found that if he rang a bell at the same time as giving food to dogs, the dogs began to associate the ringing of the bell with food. As time passed, the dogs began to salivate at the sound of the bell even in the absence of food; this demonstrated a conditioned response

Source: Adapted from Wild (2014).

Behaviourism

This is a theory that was made popular by Skinner, an American behavioural psychologist in the 1940s, and Pavlov, a Russian psychologist in the 1960s. If a repeated incentive, positive or negative, for example, an electric shock or the provision of food, is used often enough to reward or punish, then ultimately the subject will learn. These theories are associated with 'conditioned response' and 'operant conditioning' (see table 10.3).

van Vonderen (2004) suggests that behaviourist learning orientation is particularly useful when developing competencies and for demonstrating technical or psychomotor skills. This approach is most useful when a change in behaviour is the anticipated outcome of an educational intervention, and hence its popularity in health care education (Rostami and Khadjooi, 2010).

Within the health care arena Joseph et al. (1992) note that it is important that students receive immediate corrective feedback concerning incorrect concepts. Receiving feedback and expecting this to be taken on board in some circumstances will only work if it is administered immediately after performance of behaviour.

Humanism

This theory focuses on the individual. Within the humanist framework, learning is seen as a personal act that is necessary to achieve the learner's full potential. The aim of this approach is for the learner to become autonomous and self-directed. Humanist activities facilitate collaborative learning with a strong emphasis on learners and instructors discussing objectives, methods and the criteria that will evaluate outcomes (Lown et al., 2007); humanism engages the learner in an intense and personal way. The nurse helps the learner to identify individual learner-centred objectives that are drawn from experience. The emphasis is on individual responsibility for learning; according to Scanlon (2006), this is underpinned by the learner's motivation to learn and is driven by a craving to become all that he or she is capable of becoming.

Rostami and Khadjooi (2010) suggest there are five basic objectives of the humanistic view of education:

1 Promote positive self-direction and independence.
2 Develop the ability to take responsibility for what is learned.
3 Develop creativity and different ways of thinking.
4 Encourage curiosity.
5 Develop the affective/emotional elements of the learner.

Theories of learning form much of the educational content of mentorship modules. These modules are designed to facilitate nurses to develop, explore and apply the principles of teaching, learning and assessing in the practice settings. They tend to focus on developing and maintaining supportive learning environments, learning theories and learning styles, principles and processes of assessment in clinical practice, role-modelled learning and developing innovation in the practice setting.

When working with other adults in teaching in the clinical environment the nurse needs to consider the specific needs of the adult learner. Andragogy and pedagogy are two approaches to learning that should be taken into account when teaching adults in the clinical setting.

Adult learning

Knowles in the 1970s defined the term andragogy as 'an emerging technology for adult learning'; he suggested that the methods used to teach children (pedagogy) are often not the most effective ways of teaching adults (Knowles et al., 2011) (see table 10.4).

Knowles et al. (2011) derived four andragogical assumptions about adults and their learning suggesting that they:

1 Move from dependency to self-directedness
2 Draw upon their reservoir of experience for learning
3 Are ready to learn when they assume new roles
4 Want to solve problems and apply new knowledge immediately.

Andragogy claims the adult learns best when:

- They feel the need to learn
- They have some input into what, why and how it is they learn
- The learning content and processes have a meaningful relationship to the learner's past experience

Table 10.4 Pedagogy and andragogy.

Pedagogy – the methods and practices used in teaching children	Andragogy – the methods and practices used usually in teaching adults
The focus is on the teacher's methods of transferring knowledge to a student, who is dependent on the teacher's methods and understanding	The emphasis is on independent, self-directed and/or cooperative learning among adults
Teacher controls the learning experience, and much of what is taught is based on rigid guidelines	Adults have control over much of their learning experience; they must be motivated to learn. The learning often seeks out new or different learning experiences, at will

Source: Adapted from Knowles et al. (2011).

- Their experience is used as a learning resource
- What is to be learned relates to the person's current life situation
- They have as much autonomy as possible
- The learning environment minimises anxiety and encourages freedom to experiment
- Their own learning style is taken into account.

(Adapted from Quinn and Hughes (2013))

When preparing to teach the nurse should take the factors discussed earlier into account. Wild (2014) suggests that five steps should be used as a framework to help with teaching in the clinical environment:

1 Create a positive learning environment.
2 Know who your learners are.
3 Know what it is that you want them to know.
4 Prepare for the session.
5 Request feedback.

While your expertise is the key resource to be used in the teaching of learners there are a number of other human and material resources that can and should be used (see table 10.5).

Providing feedback to students

Students learn from feedback (and this should also be considered as feed-forward) but only if this is provided in a constructive manner. There may be times when feedback has to be immediate and you may need to intervene to protect the patient and the student from a potentially hazardous or undesirable procedure.

Table 10.5 Some human and material resources that can be used when teaching learners in the clinical setting.

- Use practice placement assessment documents
- Use human resources available, that is, other members of the multidisciplinary team
- Patients and families
- Case note
- Care plans
- Institutional action plans
- Outcomes of adverse reports
- Individual placement objectives
- Evidence-based practice article
- Knowledge of local/national policies, procedures and protocols

---

Over to you staff nurse

You are working with two second year student nurses and a rare event has occurred; you have an hour available to provide a teaching session for these students on the administration of an intra muscular injection.

What do you need to know prior to undertaking the teaching session?
What do you need to do prior to undertaking the teaching session?
How do you prepare for this session?
How do you evaluate your performance?
How do you give feedback to the students on their performance?

Duffy (2013) discusses the need to provide students with regular feedback on their performance as key to the assessment process. Feedback is a central aspect of the educational process for students and can aid learning. Performance-based feedback allows for good habits to be reinforced and for faulty habits to be corrected. Despite its importance, many students do not feel that they receive adequate and effective feedback. By using a straightforward and practical approach the nurse can offer the student feedback they can use to develop further.

Even the most experienced teachers can find it a challenge to provide effective feedback to learners. Anything that helps the learner to see feedback for what it really is – an informed, non-evaluative, objective appraisal of performance that is intended to improve clinical skills, as opposed to a subjective guess or estimate of a learner's personal worth – will help the process. Often, there is a mismatch between the teachers' and learners' perceptions of the purpose of the task and this is why it is important to be clear on what it is you are expecting from the student and how and where feedback will be given.

Things to think about

Feedback

Feedback should be:
- Undertaken with the nurse and learner working as allies, with common goals
- Well thought about and expected (not unexpected and ad hoc)
- Based on primary data and not hearsay
- Regulated in quantity and limited to behaviours that are remediable
- Phrased in a descriptive language
- Addressing specific performance, not generalisations
- Dealing with decisions and actions, as opposed to assumed intentions or interpretations.

Involving patients in clinical teaching

Patients are used a great deal for teaching learners, as nursing takes place in the workplace. There are many ways patients can be involved in clinical teaching. Experiential learning is a crucial component in teaching clinical and communication skills to students. However, there are a number of challenges that arise from patient involvement in health care education. Spencer et al. (2011) suggest that these range from practical considerations concerning the organisation of clinical placements to patient concerns regarding consent and confidentiality. Addressing these challenges requires the nurse to be flexible and provide innovative solutions.

Consent and confidentiality are major concerns for patients and carers when involved in teaching (Spencer et al., 2011). These issues can be addressed by appropriate preparation and orientation: the nurse should clearly explain the purpose and importance of their involvement, gain informed consent, limit health information provided to students to what is necessary to their learning and ensuring strict guidelines about confidentiality (NMC, 2015). The nurse must also be alert to the potential for exploitation of people's goodwill.

Simulation is another way that students can learn along with online teaching and learning packages. Using this approach requires the student to be very much self-directed as it requires motivation and engagement with the materials.

Patient teaching

Effective patient teaching has the potential to improve outcomes and may even save lives. Quality patient teaching requires the nurse to provide education during every encounter they have with patients and their families. The reader is advised to delve deeper into this subject area and support their understanding by accessing the literature.

The NMC (2015) make it quite clear that the provision of information related to patient teaching is a central aspect of the nurse's role. Understanding and having an awareness of the various teaching theories discussed earlier will ensure that you recognise what it is that an adult learner requires, the skills that you will have to utilise in teaching situations with the intention of helping the person to take some or more control over their health and well-being (Lappin, 2014).

Things to think about

Patient teaching

Le May (2015) suggests the basic principles of educating someone about health issues:
- Determine what it is the person needs to know.
- Work out what the person already knows.
- Work out the best ways to fill the gaps, if there are any; begin from where the person is.
- When people are ill or uncomfortable or anxious, their concentration levels may be poor.
- Be clear and concise in what it is you are saying; always use easy, simple to follow language.
- Provide information in small bite-size chunks and check that the person has understood what you have said.
- Remember to supplement verbal information provided with written information.
- Always tell a person where he or she can seek further advice should he or she forget what it is you have said.
- If possible, set up with the patient another meeting to check out what he or she has heard and leant and how he or she is using the information you have given.
- Involve the family if the patient agrees to this.

Conclusion

Effective education empowers, be this effective nurse education or effective patient education. This chapter has outlined the role of the newly qualified nurse as a teacher and has referred to the NMC's (2008) developmental stages. Acting as a stage 1 teacher is expected as soon as the nurse registers with the NMC and stage 2 teacher status can be attained after successful completion of an NMC-approved programme of study of one year's post-qualification.

Teaching and learning in the clinical setting occurs across a range of diverse environments, frequently in widely spread locations, in the National Health Service and elsewhere in the public, independent and voluntary sectors. It is a demanding and complex task that many nurses assume without adequate preparation or orientation. Several roles have been described for those who teach in the clinical environment.

The learning environment should enable students to develop competence in order to become safe, caring, competent, knowledgeable decision-makers who understand personal and professional accountability for care that they provide. The clinical practice experience forms the central focus of the profession and is a key component of the pre-registration nurse education programme.

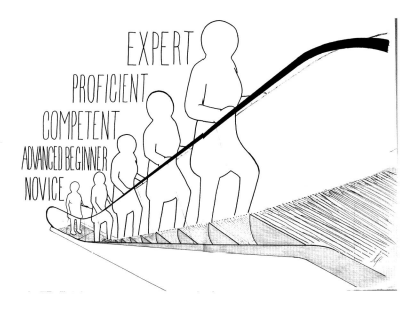

There are varieties of theories of learning at the nurse's disposal; it is essential to identify the principles of learning and to understand how individual differences can influence the learning process. Behaviourism and humanism are two such theories.

Adult learning and the methods used to teach adults (andragogy) differ from those used to teach children (pedagogy). Understanding the difference in these approaches can help the nurse structure clinical teaching to meet the needs of the student.

Involving patients in clinical teaching can enhance the learning experience; experiential learning is a central component in teaching clinical and communication skills to students. However, there are some challenges that may arise when using this approach, such as consent and confidentiality. Addressing these issues demands that the nurse be flexible and innovative.

References

An Bord Altranais (2003) "Guidelines on the Key Points That May be Considered When Developing a Quality Clinical Learning Environment". An Bord Altranais: Dublin.

Barton, D. and Le May, A. (2012) "Adult Nursing. Preparing for Practice". Hodder and Arnold: London.

Duffy, K. (2013) "Providing Constructive Feedback to Students During Mentorship". Nursing Standard, Vol 27, No 31, pp. 50–56.

Emmanuel, V. and Pryce-Miler, M. (2013) "Creating Supportive Environments for Students". Nursing Times, Vol 109, No **37**, pp. 19–20.

Harden, R.M. and Crosby, J.R. (2000) "AMEE Guide No 20: The Good Teacher is More Than a Lecturer: The Twelve Roles of the Teacher". Medical Teacher, Vol 22, pp. 334–347.

Joseph, A., Abraham, S., Bhattacharji, S., Muliyil, J., John, K.R., Ethirajan, N., et al. (1992) "The Teaching of Behavioural Sciences". Medical Education, Vol 26, pp. 92–98.

Kinnell, D. and Hughes, P. (2010) "Mentoring Nursing and Healthcare Students". Sage: London.

Knowles, M., Horton, E.E. and Swanson, R.E. (2011) (11th Ed) "The Adult Learner: The Definitive Classic in Adult Education and Human Resource Development". Butterworth: Oxford.

Kolb, D. A. (1984) "Experiential Learning: Experience as the Source of Learning and Development". Prentice Hall: New Jersey.

Lappin, M. (2014) "Models of Nursing", in Peate, I., Wild, K. and Nair, M. (Eds) "Nursing Practice and Knowledge", Ch 7, pp. 130–146. Wiley: Oxford.

Le May, A. (2015) "Adult Nursing at a Glance". Wiley: Oxford.

Lown, B.A., Chou, C.L., Clark, W.D., Haidet, P., White, M.K., Krupat, E., et al. (2007) "Caring Attitudes in Medical Education: Perceptions of Deans and Curriculum Leaders". Journal of General Internal Medicine, Vol 22, pp. 1514–1522.

Nursing and Midwifery Council (2008) (2nd Ed) "Standards to Support Learning and Assessment in Practice". NMC: London.

Nursing and Midwifery Council (2010) "Standards for Pre Registrations Nurse Education" http://standards.nmc-uk.org/PublishedDocuments/Standards%20for%20pre-registration%20nursing%20education%2016082010.pdf last (accessed February 2015).

Nursing and Midwifery Council (2015) "The Code. Professional Standards of Practice and Behaviour for Nurses and Midwives" http://www.nmc-uk.org/Documents/NMC-Publications/NMC-Code-A5-FINAL.pdf last (accessed February 2015).

Papp, M., Markkanen, M. and von Bondsdorff, M. (2003) "Clinical Environment as a Learning Environment: Student Nurses' Perceptions Concerning Clinical Learning Environment". Nurse Education Today, Vol 23, No **4**, pp. 262–267.

Quinn, F.M. and Hughes, S.J. (6th Ed) (2013) "Quinn's Principles and Practice of Nurse Education". Cengage Learning: Andover.

Rostami, K. and Khadjooi, K. (2010) "The Implications of Behaviorism and Humanism Theories in Medical Education". Gastroenterology and Hepatology From Bed to Bench, Vol 3, No **2**, pp. 65–70.

Scanlon, A. (2006) "Humanistic Principles in Relation to Psychiatric Nurse Education: A Review of the Literature". Journal of Psychiatric Mental Health Nursing, Vol 13, pp. 758–764.

Schon, D.A. (1987) "Educating the Reflective Practitioner". Jossey-Bass: San Francisco.

Spencer, J., Godolphin, W., Karpenko, N., Towle, A. (2011) "Can Patients be Teachers? Involving Patients and Service Users in Healthcare Professionals' Education". The Health Foundation: Newcastle.

van Vonderen, A. (2004) "Effectiveness of Immediate Verbal Feedback on Trainer Behaviour During Communication Training with Individuals with Intellectual Disability". Journal of Intellectual Disability Research, Vol 48, pp. 245–251.

Wild, K. (2014) "The Professional Nurse and Contemporary Health Care", in Peate, I., Wild, K. and Nair, M. (Eds) "Nursing Practice and Knowledge" Ch 2, pp. 25–49. Wiley: Oxford.

Index

Note: Page numbers in *italic* refer to figures and tables
Page numbers in **bold** refer to definitions

A

abdominal surgery, evidence-based practice, 86
accountability, 22, 40, 52, 58, **64**, 72–3
  advanced nurse practitioners, 108
  contracts of employment, 61
  legal, 61
  NHS, 93
  NMC *Code of Conduct*, 60–1, 65
  and responsibility, 58–60
  spheres of, *60*
  teaching roles, 169
  see also delegation; supervision of others
accredited advanced nursing practice programmes, 117
activities required as part of training
  continuing professional development, *162*, 162–3
  new nurses, *56*
adult learning (andragogy), 177–8, *178*, **178**, 182
advanced beginners stage of clinical competence, *110*, 111
advanced nurse practitioners, 107–8, 122–3
  accountability and responsibility, 108
  assessment, *119*
  careers, 28, *29–30*
  inter-relationships, *109*
  job titles and terminology, 114–17
  prescribing, 107, 110, *118*, 120–2
  professional indemnity, 119–20
  pros and cons, 118
  stages of clinical competence, *110*, 110–14
  standards, 108, 109–10
  training towards, 117–19, *118*, *119*
Agenda for Change pay scheme, 34

andragogy, 177–8, *178*, **178**, 182
anecdotal evidence, 81
anger, emotional phases of change, *139*
annual appraisals, 153–4
application forms for jobs, 2, 8–10, *9*
appraisal, professional development, 151–7, **152**, *153*, *154*
apps, medical, 39
aptitude tests, psychometric testing, 12–13
assessment
  advanced nurse practitioners, *119*
  preceptorship, 50–1
assessment of patient needs, delegation, 65–7
assistant practitioners, *3*
assumptions, challenging, 76
audits, clinical, 78, *129*, *162*

B

bargaining, emotional phases of change, *139*
barriers to change
  change management, *140*, 140
  evidence-based practice, 85–7, *86*
behaviourism, 176, *176*
bowel sounds, evidence-based practice, 86
breast cancer, evidence-based practice, 83
bullying at work, 138

C

care interventions, evidence-based practice, 84–5
Care Quality Commission (CQC), 79, 85
Career Framework for Health, NHS, 34–5
careers in nursing, 1–2, 27, 40
  career goals, 38, 40
  core dimensions of nursing, *35*, *36*
  developing the role, 37–40
  frameworks, 30–2, *31*, 34–5
  job descriptions, 35–6
  modernising, 27–8, *29–30*, 115. *see also* advanced nurse practitioners

---

The Essential Guide to Becoming a Staff Nurse, First Edition. Ian Peate.
© 2016 John Wiley & Sons, Ltd. Published 2016 by John Wiley & Sons, Ltd.

dignity of patients, NHS values, *94*
dimensions of nursing, KSF framework, *35, 36*
distance learning, continuing professional development, *162*
documentation
  CPD portfolios, 151, 158, *162*, 163–4, *164*, 165–6
  preceptorship, 50–1, *51*
duty of care, *37*, 66, 108

E
education, management roles, *128–9*
effectiveness and efficiency, NHS Constitution, *93*
e-learning, support systems for new nurses, *54*, 54–5
emotional phases of change, 138, *139*, 145
employee rights, 127
Equality Act (2010), 138
equilibrium, emotional phases of change, *139*
equity, NHS values, 47, *93*, *94*
European Working Time Directive (1993), 115
evidence-based practice (EBP) xii,, 33, 74–6, 87
  advanced nurse practitioners, 117
  appraisal of evidence, *83*, 83–4
  care interventions based on, 84–5
  challenges to implementation, 85–7, *86*
  clinical governance, 77–9
  decision-making based on, 84
  hierarchy of evidence, *82*
  performance evaluation, 84
  preceptorship, 46
  sources of evidence, *81*, 81–2
  stages, 79–84, *80*
expert power, *137*
expert stage of clinical competence, *110*, 111, 113–14
extended roles, 108. *see also* advanced nurse practitioners

F
feedback
  giving, 178–80
  receiving, 150, *151*, 176
Francis Report (2013), 151

G
goal-setting
  continuing professional development, 156–7
  time management, 136

guidelines
  continuing professional development, 148
  Nursing and Midwifery Council, 110
  see also standards
guiding principles, NHS Constitution, 92–4, *93*

H
harassment at work, 138
Health and Social Care Act (2012), 2–5, *4*, 27, 108
health care assistants, *3*
health care reform, xi
  and accountability, 59–60
  nursing roles, 37–8. *see also* advanced nurse practitioners
  societal changes, *33*
Health Committee, complaints procedures, 103
healthcare plans, advanced nurse practitioners, 118
HealthWatch, 4
high-level skills, staff nurse roles, 36
homeworkfor interviews, 4, 5
hours of practice, 149, *149*, 150, *164*
humanism, 176–7

I
image of nursing, modernising, 28, *29*
indemnity insurance, 119–20
induction, new nurses, 53, *54*
internet searching, 38–9
interviews, 14–18
  hints and tips, 17
  homework, 4, 5
  questions to ask, *16*
  structure, *18*
  what to wear, 18

J
job descriptions, 5–8, *6*
  advanced nurse practitioners, 108
  management roles, 127, *128–9*
  staff nurse roles, 35–6, *37*
  team working, *128–9*, 141
job hunting, 1–2, *3*, 19
  application forms, 8–10, *9*
  awareness of legislation, 2–5, *4*
  curriculum vitae, 10–12
  interviews, 4, 5, 14–18, *16*
  numeracy screening, 14
  overseas positions, 19
  personal statements, 10
  psychometric testing, 12–13